THE TESTOSTERONE EDGE

THE TESTOSTERONE EDGE

The Healthy, Safe, and Effective Way to Boost Energy, Fight Disease, and Increase Sexual Vitality

BRIAN E. O'NEILL

FOREWORD BY PETER N. SCHLEGEL, M.D., F.A.C.S.

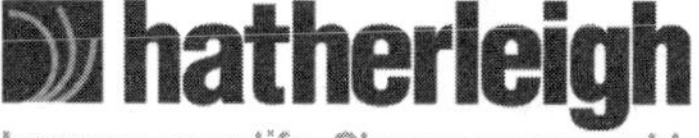

Improve your life. Change your world.
New York

Hatherleigh Press
5-22 46th Avenue, Suite 200
Long Island City, NY 11101
www.hatherleighpress.com

DISCLAIMER
This book does not give legal or medical advice. Always consult your doctor, lawyer, and other professionals. The names of people who contributed anecdotal material have been changed.

Brand names are typically followed by TM or ® symbols, but these symbols are not stated in this book.

The ideas and suggestions contained in this book are not intended as a substitute for consulting with a physician. All matters regarding your health require medical supervision.

Library of Congress Cataloging-in-Publication Data
O'Neill, Brian E.
The testosterone edge : the healthy, safe, and effective way to boost energy, fight disease, and increase sexual vitality / Brian E. O'Neill ;
foreword by Peter N. Schlegel.
p. cm.
Includes index.
ISBN 978-1-57826-253-3
1. Testosterone--Physiological effect—Popular works. I. Title.
QP572.T4O64 2007
612.6'1—dc22
2007017015

The Testosterone Edge is available for bulk purchase, special promotions, and premiums. For information on reselling and special purchase opportunities, call 1-800-528-2550 and ask for the Special Sales Manager.

Interior design by Deborah Miller and Jacinta Monniere
Cover design by Farrimond New York

10 9 8 7 6 5 4 3 2 1
Printed in the United States

This is a book about testosterone.
I dedicate it to my wife, Christine. 'Nuff said?

ACKNOWLEDGEMENTS

THERE MAY BE ONLY ONE AUTHOR OF THIS BOOK, but several other people, whether they realize it or not, deserve thanks and credit for its existence. First, I'd like to thank my parents, Richard O'Neill Sr. and Donna Ewing-Fullerton. They always told me that if I set my mind to it, I could accomplish all that I wanted to in life—and so I did. To Ron Hutson and Cheryl Appel, two editors at *The Boston Globe* who essentially began my writing career. Thanks also to Nancy Ferrari and Ed Coburn at Harvard Health Publications, who probably have no idea how much they've done to help me along in my career as a health writer.

I owe a debt of gratitude to the medical professionals who shared their knowledge, experience, and stories, and who didn't laugh at what I must assume were some pretty stupid questions. Special thanks to Dr. Harvey B. Simon from Harvard University, Dr. Tracy Wimbush from Massachusetts General Hospital, Dr. John Morley from St. Louis University, Dr. Robert Tan from the University of Texas, and Drs. Dana Cohen and Jennifer Landa (both in private practice). And of course an extra special thanks to Dr. Peter N. Schlegel from the The New York Presbyterian Hospital-Weill Cornell Medical Center for writing the foreword.

I'm also indebted to those whose specialized knowledge in areas of diet, exercise, and pharmaceuticals contributed greatly to this book. Thanks to registered dietician Lori Magrath for feedback and guidance on the diet information appearing in chapter 9. Thanks to Pavel Tsatsouline (the "evil Russian") for generous help on the exercise information in chapter 8. (Power to you, Comrade!) A tip of the hat to pharmacist Nina Patel, for comprehensive information on medical testosterone replacement therapy, as appears in chapter 6.

My deepest thanks to those who selflessly shared their personal experiences with testosterone replacement or testosterone-level difficulties: Carol Arnold, Jeff Altman, Lisa Hutchinson, and "John" (who knows who he is). Thanks to Paul Frediani for literally doing the heavy lifting with this book. His demonstrations of the exercises and stretches in chapter 8 are invaluable.

A literary high five to Andrea Au and Kevin Moran at Hatherleigh Press, for taking a chance on a young writer, and for—miraculously—finding a book within my writings. And to the all-star lineup at Hatherleigh Press responsible for buffing this book to a high sheen: assistant editor Alyssa Smith, art director/production manager Deborah Miller, and publicity associate Erin Byram.

Testosterone is, as you'll learn in the following pages, literally what makes a man a man—in the biological sense. But then there's what it means to be a man in the John Wayne sense, the do-what-you-gotta-do (even when it's the last thing you want to do) sense. And nobody has taught me more about that than my uncle, Scott Ewing. Over the last year he has faced serious challenges with a level of courage, grace, and poise that makes me feel downright silly for fretting about deadlines and word counts. I'm lucky and proud to know you, old friend.

And finally, I'd like to thank my beautiful, loving, patient wife, Christine Junge, for putting up with me while I was writing this book. And for putting up with me in general.

CONTENTS

FOREWORD

CAN A MAN HAVE TOO MUCH TESTOSTERONE? IS low testosterone (testosterone deficiency) a disease or merely a reflection of the natural aging process? Is testosterone therapy a remarkable achievement that allows men access to a fountain-of-youth-like state or a dangerous, unproven medical therapy? Even in medical circles, problems related to insufficient or excess testosterone levels are poorly understood.

Brian O'Neill presents these issues and more in this straightforward, easy-to-read, and informative book. Sorting through the myths and misinformation that surround testosterone, he uses verified medical information to explain the complex process of testosterone production and action.

Production of testosterone is almost never constant, rising in limited periods of childhood development (including the period immediately after birth), then fading into quiescence for more than a decade before raging back to effect the sexual characteristics that we identify as "male" in the rapidly evolving creature that is an adolescent young man. Testosterone drives normal libido, sexual activity, fertility and, to some degree, creativity. It also supports some of the more outrageous behaviors that we see in our society.

The prevalent abuse of androgens (male hormones) in the form of synthetic steroids is a reflection both of how much testosterone action is desired by men, and how closely related testosterone action is to our view of what is "male." For young men to risk shrinkage of their testes, liver tumors, infertility, and other medical complications with the persistent abuse of anabolic steroids is almost inconceivable until one considers the powerful sway of "virility" in our culture.

The progressive decrease in a man's production of testosterone with aging is dramatic, especially as men enter their seventh decade and beyond. The remarkable improvements in well-being, muscle mass, thought processes, and sexual function attributed to testosterone therapy are even more dramatic. However, we lack a clear dividing line between what is normal in testosterone production and action and what is not. In addition, little scientific data exists to identify which patients are most likely to benefit from testosterone treatment and whether there are long-term medical risks from such treatment.

This medical uncertainty has recently been tempered with "Consensus Guidelines" that give physicians information on how to guide patients with concerns about low testosterone levels. These guidelines, combining the American Society for Reproductive Medicine (ASRM) Practice Guidelines and the Endocrine Society's Concensus Panel Report on how to evaluate and treat men with low testosterone levels, were written and developed based on a review of existent published medical literature by a panel of medical experts in the field. They represent the combined view of specialists who care for men with low testosterone levels, and I am glad I was able to play a part in preparing these guidelines as the urologist on the ASRM Practice Committee.

The treatment of low testosterone levels is a controversial medical field that carries both promise and peril for men and women. Because conflicting information exists, patients may be led to expect more benefits of treatment than are likely to occur, or they might miss the possibility that low testosterone levels is responsible for their symptoms. This book helps them understand how testosterone works, and whether evaluation and treatment could be worthwhile for them. In addition, it provides clear and extensive information on the potential side effects of hormone treatments they may be suggested by their physician.

I hope you find the book as readable—and as useful—as I have. I will certainly be recommending the book to my patients.

Peter N. Schlegel, M.D., F.A.C.S.
Professor & Chairman
Department of Urology
Weill Medical College of Cornell University
New York Presbyterian Hospital

Introduction

In 2001 a young police officer checked himself into the emergency room at a local hospital in the middle of the night, bleeding and considerably weakened. His breath was heavy and labored, while a profuse sweat covered his face and body. He had the frail, gaunt look of a man three times his age. As the doctors crowded around him they were able to stop the bleeding, but the harm may have been permanent: his liver had been hit hard and badly damaged.

Had he been shot or stabbed in the line of duty? Had he suffered injuries in a car crash resulting from a high-speed chase?

No. He had been abusing synthetic testosterone, better known as anabolic steroids.

The bleeding was due to the abscesses on his arms at the injection sites. The liver damage was due to the damaging effects of a tidal surge of a hormone that the body produces in only relatively small amounts. The officer had been abusing steroids since 1993, and was 27 at the time of his first hospital visit—but he looked like he was an unhealthy 65.

Doctors eventually had to put him on a respirator and perform surgery to remove blood clots and to attempt to repair his liver. They were stunned that a young, strong, and seemingly intelligent man could be so dramatically weakened by the very hormone associated with strength and virility. They were even more stunned when he came back to the emergency room nine months later with the same problems, due to continued abuse. Massive amounts of testosterone had had the precise opposite effect to what he had expected.

You don't need to abuse steroids to get swept up in our national obsession with testosterone. It doesn't take much more than a daily sweep of unsolicited e-mails to know that supplements, gadgets, and gizmos guaranteeing higher testosterone levels have flooded the Internet marketplace and health-food store shelves. It doesn't take a Sherlock Holmes to deduce that it's pretty suspicious that so many records have been broken in professional sports over the last two decades. You don't even need to be an athlete or body builder to know that testosterone is responsible for muscle mass, libido, bone strength, mood, and more.

But many men may not realize that the very chemical essence of their manhood is produced in increasingly short supply with each passing year after about age 30. It is the physiological destiny of every man on this planet to have less and less testosterone as the years go by, sometimes—but not always—culminating in an array of unpleasant symptoms. Hence, the quest for restoring or maintaining a lean and muscular body and a youthful sex drive throughout life.

I wrote this book primarily for men who want to know more about testosterone and make informed decisions about how, if at all, to address the natural decline that accompanies normal, healthy aging. Along the way, we'll explore the many myths, lies, and cover-ups associated with testosterone replacement, supplements, steroids, and wacked-out claims with regard to how a man can increase his testosterone naturally.

I've done the best I can to arrange the material in this book in a logical and consistent manner. In chapter 1 we'll take a look at exactly what testosterone is and does, and how the body produces it. Chapter 2 explores the effects and symptoms of testosterone when it is in too-short supply, as well as when there's too much (the above story ought to give you an idea). Chapters 3 and 4 take a look at the connection between testosterone and overall health. We'll look at health conditions that can have a lowering effect on testosterone, as well as health conditions that may themselves be the result of too much or too little testosterone. In chapter 5, we debate whether there is indeed such a thing as "male menopause" that results from the symptoms of flagging hormone levels at the beginning of middle age. Part 2 of this book explores treatment options, medical, non-medical, and even downright silly. We'll weigh the pros and cons of medical testosterone replacement therapy, take an inside look at supplements that claim to boost testosterone (or at least replicate some of the effects of the hormone), and learn how diet and exercise can promote many of the same rejuvenating effects—without drugs or gimmicky supplements.

Finally, we'll address testosterone as it pertains to women—yes, women. (And I'm not just talking about how *your* testosterone-fueled sex drive affects your poor wife.) Albeit in comparatively miniscule amounts, the female body also creates testosterone, for largely the same reason a man's body does—and with similar effects and symptoms when production drops off for any number of reasons.

Though the content builds on itself from chapter to chapter, you're free to dive into any particular chapter that catches your interest. You'll notice at the end of each chapter that I've highlighted the main points in a section called "The Low-Down," which ought to give you a good idea of what's covered, and also to serve as a review when you've finished reading each chapter.

Overall, my goal is to provide you with the most up-to-date information available today, and present controversial topics as objectively as possible. In the end, it is up to you and your doctor to manage and address all aspects of your health and well-being, including your testosterone levels.

PART I

UNDERSTANDING TESTOSTERONE

IN THE PAGES THAT FOLLOW WE'RE GOING TO TAKE the first steps toward understanding what—chemically speaking, at least—it means to be a healthy man. Let's call it an owner's manual for this potent little hormone we know and love as testosterone. Some of what you read may surprise you or contradict what you thought you already knew. Some of it will be old hat. So be it. Getting *The Testosterone Edge* means first laying a solid foundation of knowledge and understanding on which we'll build subsequent ideas and theories. You may be tempted to skip over some of the material in the following chapters. My advice: don't. If you want to dive into the more "exciting" material first, that's fine, but make sure you come back to chapters 1 to 5 before you begin on any of the program material you find in this book. You wouldn't build a house without a blueprint. You wouldn't bake a cake without a cookbook. And you won't get *The Testosterone Edge* without a rudimentary understanding of the basic information of what testosterone is and does, and how and why it's produced.

If you're ready to begin, I'm ready to guide you. Turn the page, and let's get started.

CHAPTER 1:

WHAT IS TESTOSTERONE?

IF EVER THERE WERE A HUMAN HORMONE TO ACHIEVE "rock star" status, no doubt it would be our old friend testosterone. You could say it's got a reputation. If you could buy it a drink, you gladly would—and it would unquestionably be a beer (nay, a "brewskie"). It's become a code word for virility, manliness, and attractiveness. It's also become a code word for lunk-headedness. Certain behaviors and personality qualities commonly considered exclusively male, including competitiveness, stoicism, aggressiveness, ambitiousness, egotism, thrill-seeking, and assertiveness, are routinely traced back to testosterone in the court of public opinion. The guy who paints himself red and goes shirtless to a football game? Blame it on the T. The gym rat who can't help but grunt and groan and flex for himself in the mirror? Must be high on testosterone. Highway speeding, libidinous barroom antics, corporate backstabbing—testosterone was there without an excuse, the potion that turns Jekyll into Hyde.

Never has hormone become so deeply ingrained in our vocabulary, and become so closely associated—whether fairly or correctly or not—with just about all things male. Action adventure movies are often billed as "testosterone-fueled." Loud, hard-core music is advertised as "testosterized." On an episode of *Friends,* Phoebe accused Joey of being "testosteroney" for not wanting to call a woman back after their first date. Open your local newspaper and take a gander at the headlines. On a recent week I found no fewer than 25 headlines equating the mighty T with what is often passed off as "male behavior." *Seattle Times* editorial writer Collin Levey, criticizing then-presidential candidate John Kerry's attempts at "guy's guy" behavior, proclaimed that "It's About Terrorism, John, Not Testosterone Levels."[1]

Testosterone has been called the hormone of desire, not referring to just sexual desire, but all kinds of desire. In an episode of the National Public Radio program *This American Life,* a man told of an experience where, due to a medical condition, his body stopped producing testosterone, and he was without it for several months. In his account of that experience, he remembered:

> "When you have no testosterone you have no desire and...you don't think about anything. I was...sitting in bed staring at the wall, with neither interest nor disinterest, for three, four hours at a time. If you had had a camera in the room, you'd have thought I was comatose...I had no interest in watching TV, much less reading a book. People who are deprived of testosterone don't become 'Spock-like' and incredibly rational; they become nonsensical, because they're unable to distinguish between what is, and isn't, interesting."[2]

Our obsession with testosterone is actually nothing new, far from it. More than 100 years ago many men subscribed to the idea that overall aging, including a decline in sex drive and sexual performance was connected to a drop in "male factors." A popular "therapy" emerged in the health spas frequented by the wealthy, where extracts from the testicles of farm animals were injected daily into the men's rear ends.[3] The developer of the therapy, a French physiologist named Charles Édouard Brown-Séquard (who was later credited as being one of the fathers of modern endocrinology) claimed that his "liquide testiculair" increased his physical strength and—oddly enough—lengthened the arc of his urine.

Say it with me now: "Ewwww!" Not only is it gross, but the basic idea is way, way off. Testosterone, as we're about to discuss, is *produced* in the testes, but not *stored* there. In fact, there was no more testosterone in that "liquide" than there would have been had the good doctor extracted from any other part of any animal's body. Thank goodness such a useless (and probably dangerous) practice is no longer *en vogue*, but we're not exactly out of the woods yet. Cruise the vitamin aisle at your local drugstore for any number of over-the-counter items making some pretty outrageous claims based on some pretty suspicious ingredients. We'll talk in much more detail about supplements in chapter 7.

Our understanding of testosterone is still very much in its infancy, and because of the glut of information and misinformation out there—in popular bodybuilding and men's interest magazines, movies, and the pharmaceuticals market—the myth machine keeps on cranking. Today, there are nine testosterone myths, rumors, and lies that lead the pack:

1. **Myth: Only men need to be concerned about testosterone levels.** Sorry, ladies. The female body produces a small, but not insignificant, amount of testosterone, which can have undesired effects when diminished, including a significant drop in libido. Many menopausal women receive testosterone replacement therapy (usually through a topical gel or patch) to help restore the decreased sex drive that sometimes follows menopause. Likewise, certain medical conditions such as polycystic ovarian syndrome are consistent with elevated levels of testosterone, which also can produce undesired effects, such as facial hair growth, a deepened voice, and male-pattern-style balding, among others. We will discuss these and other issues in chapters 11 and 12.
2. **Myth: Low testosterone affects only older men.** Wrong again. While the average man will begin to see a steady decline beginning in his early thirties (with the effects becoming noticeable by his mid forties), the truth is that low testosterone can come at just about any age. In chapter 3 we'll discuss some of the ways that low testosterone can affect young men—even infants.
3. **Myth: Testosterone is necessary for sexual function.** Sort of. Testosterone has relatively little to do with the physical processes that result in the ability to perform sexually—to achieve and maintain an erection. A man with almost nonexistent testosterone could produce an erection if given one of the popular drugs used to treat erectile dysfunction. However, increased testosterone is associated with increased libido, which is in turn associated with increased frequency of erections. (Indeed, as we'll discuss shortly, testosterone levels are highest in the morning, which helps to explain why most men wake up in a state of sexual arousal.) Therefore, decreased testosterone all but surely results in decreased libido and decreased frequency of erections. But in the end, testosterone is part of the catalyst—the things that set the stage for a man's body to produce an erection—

and not the primary mechanism. It's useful, and it's definitely desirable, but it's not essential for sexual performance.

4. **Myth: Testosterone replacement therapy improves fertility.** A popular myth, but a myth just the same. Strange that the hormone so intimately associated with virility and studliness has relatively little to do with fertility. The seminiferous tubules of the testes require testosterone (among several other things) to be present in order for them to produce sperm. And of course, an integral part of fertility is the ability to fertilize (i.e., to perform sexually), so in those respects, testosterone does play a part. When it comes to signaling the body's sperm-producing assembly line, though, it's not testosterone but a hormone produced in the brain (which we'll discuss shortly) that's most important. Testosterone replacement therapy isn't likely to be part of the treatment program for men with fertility problems. In fact, in chapter 6 we'll meet "John," a man who is on testosterone replacement therapy, but who, on the advice of his doctor, has stopped taking it in order to *improve* his chances of conception.
5. **Myth: Testosterone replacement therapy "cures" low testosterone.** Not so fast. First of all, low testosterone isn't necessarily a "disease" needing a cure, no matter what the pharmaceutical companies tell you. Secondly, testosterone replacement is a therapeutic measure, meaning that if you take it, you take it for the rest of your life. (One exception, however, is in the case of a teenage boy with abnormally delayed development, who might receive testosterone replacement therapy for a short period to induce puberty.) Problem is, as we'll discuss in chapter 6, we still don't know nearly enough to determine whether long-term (even lifelong) testosterone therapy is safe and effective.
6. **Myth: Women who receive testosterone replacement therapy will grow facial hair.** Yes, excessively high levels of testosterone in women can promote the formation of male-style cosmetic changes, including unwanted facial and body hair, male-pattern-style baldness, acne, a deepened voice, and others. But excessively high levels are not what testosterone replacement therapy for women is all about. The vast majority of women on testosterone replacement therapy will see no unwanted cosmetic changes at all.

7. **Myth: Testosterone "plummets" with age.** Nope. It declines steadily, and the decline is highly variable from one man to another. An average healthy man will start to see a decline beginning in his early 30s, which will continue at a pace of about one percent per year. That means that by age 70, he will still have about 60 percent of the testosterone levels he had at his peak. Sure, that may not be much to brag about, but it's a sufficiently high level to explain why men are often able to remain sexually active—or at least have an interest in sex or sexual activity—well into old age.
8. **Myth: Testosterone replacement therapy causes prostate cancer.** Perhaps the most pervasive myth in these days of wildly popular testosterone replacement among men. Long-term, high-dose replacement therapy is often linked to an enlargement of the prostate, which makes sense: testosterone is, after all, responsible for the growth of the prostate during puberty. These cases of enlargement during replacement therapy are rare and not fully understood, but no research to date has proven a direct connection between testosterone replacement and prostate cancer.
9. **Myth: Testosterone is what makes men more aggressive and violent than women are.** Now is that a very nice thing to say about testosterone? We'll discuss this idea in detail at the end of this chapter. Testosterone, like all hormones, plays some part in our behavior. And yes, aggressive behaviors tend to rise and fall with testosterone levels. However, this is an exceedingly short-sighted view of what is a much, much larger picture.

Testosterone, the "Man-Maker"

Whether testosterone deserves its reputation as the bad boy of the hormonal world is a debate we'll pick up later on this chapter. For now, though, let's take a look at the facts. Just what is testosterone?

First things first. Testosterone is a special kind of hormone called an androgen: "andro" from the Greek for "man," "gen," from the Latin "genitus," to beget. Literally, an androgen is a "man-maker," more commonly referred to as a "male sex hormone." But don't let the name fool you. As I mentioned, women have testosterone too, albeit in much smaller amounts. (And likewise, the male body contains very small amounts of the female equivalent of an androgen: estrogen.) There are other kinds of androgens, including dehydrotestosterone, dehydroepiandrosterone, and androstenedione (all of which we'll discuss later on), but testosterone is without question king of the mountain.

It's also classified as a steroid hormone, others of which include estrogen. There's no reason to get too heavily into the technical details, but officially, testosterone, like all steroid hormones, is based on a structure of three hexane (6 carbon) rings and one pentane (5 carbon) ring.

Testosterone begins its life as cholesterol, a form of lipid (fat) produced by the body, mainly the liver, and also taken in from some of the foods we eat. From there, cholesterol is converted to a hormone called pregnenolone, which in turn is converted into either dehydroepiandrosterone or progesterone. Progesterone is converted to androstenedione before finally becoming testosterone, and dehydroepiandrosterone spends some time as androstenediol before being further converted into testosterone. Whatever intermediary steps it takes before claiming its throne as the Mighty T are inconsequential. It's the end result that matters: testosterone is testosterone. From there, the newly made testosterone is dispatched to work its magic on the various androgen receptors of the body.

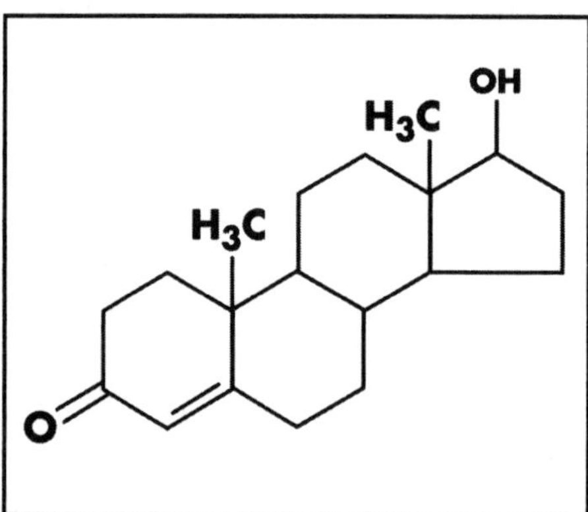

The molecular structure of testosterone.

All right, enough with the technical terminology for the moment. A bit of technical understanding can never hurt, but our goal here is to gain a general understanding of what testosterone is and does. You might be surprised by what we discuss next. While testosterone is a "man-making" substance, your body has been using it since before you were anything resembling a man—way before. Let's take a look.

Development of the Male Fetus

Believe it or not, you got your first taste of testosterone before you were even born. Testosterone is literally what makes you a man, and so it makes sense that it would play an important role in the proper development of a male fetus. In fact, at about the seventh week of development, hormones from the placenta of a mother whose fetus displays a Y chromosome trigger the production of testosterone in what will become the "Leydig cells" (named after the doctor who discovered them) of the fetus's developing testicles.

It also plays a role in the development of the brain in a way that may explain (in part, at least) certain male cognitive and behavioral traits. In the womb, testosterone appears to slow the growth of the left hemisphere of the brain, commonly associated with language and verbal expression, and enhances growth of the right hemisphere, largely responsible for spatial intelligence.[4]

Testosterone stays in production through fetal development and into a short period of infancy, and then remains largely dormant until adolescence. It is then that production kicks into high gear and sets in motion all of the processes that make the male body what it is. But before we talk about all of the wonderful ways in which testosterone makes men undeniably male, let's take a peek at the complex inner workings of the body's testosterone production machine. We're going inside the testosterone factory.

Inside the Testosterone Factory

Suppose that I'm a mad scientist on a mission to whip up a batch of testosterone. I have a full set of working human body parts at my disposal in my diabolical laboratory. Where should I begin my dirty work?

Let's recall that testosterone is a hormone, specifically, an androgen. A hormone (from the Greek "hormo," to set in motion) is a kind of chemical messenger responsible for stimulating certain activities in the various tissues of the body. Most hormones are produced by the glands of the body's endocrine system, including the pituitary (in the brain), the thyroid (near the collarbones), the adrenals (sitting atop the kidneys), and—in the case of testosterone—the testicles. That is, after all, where testosterone gets its name.

A very small amount (about 5% or so) is produced by the adrenal glands, and in women, what little is produced comes from the adrenals and ovaries. But in my laboratory, I'm going for the highest returns: I'll need to start with a working pair of testes. Heck, even one would get the job done, as Lance Armstrong could probably tell you, but I'll go with two.

Next, we'll need a switch that "turns on" the testicles' ability to begin testosterone production. For that, we'll need to travel north, all the way up to the center of the brain. The hypothalamus, located near the pituitary gland in the middle base of the brain, is wired up to the endocrine system (among other things), and is responsible for producing something called gonadotropin releasing hormone, or GnRH for short. Remember that hormones are responsible for stimulating activity in certain tissues in the body. GnRH has a solitary mission: to travel the short distance to the pituitary gland, and tell it to produce follicle-stimulating hormone (FSH) and luteinizing hormone (LH). FSH stimulates sperm production, and so it's not terribly important for our discussion. It's the LH that carries the baton in this body-wide relay race to create some testosterone.

Our newly formed LH makes its way down to the testicles, where it then commands the specialized Leydig cells to start producing testosterone.

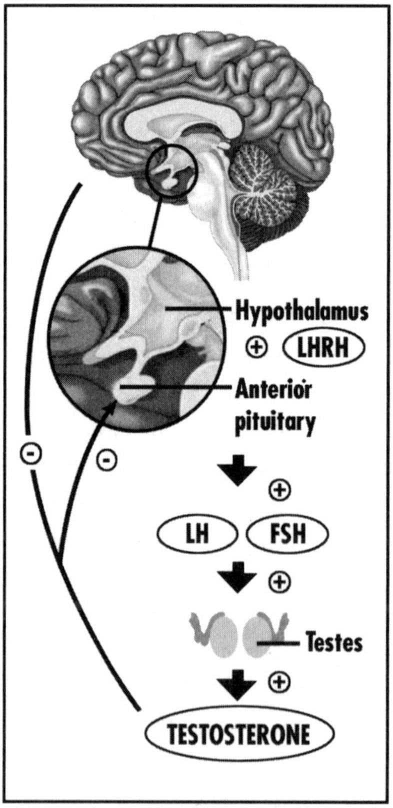

The hypothalamus-gonadal-pituitary axis: the network between the brain and the testes that produces testosterone.

'Round the Clock Production

Like most major biological functions, your body's production of testosterone follows a predictable 24-hour cycle known as a "circadian rhythm." Circadian rhythms, including alertness levels, core body temperature, and digestive function naturally rise and fall throughout the day, governed by a small cluster of cells in the brain known as the "suprachiasmatic nucleus" or "body clock."

When it comes to testosterone, production is at its peak in the early morning. This should be obvious to most men (especially young men), for whom waking up in a state of physical sexual arousal is the norm. Production drops sharply after early

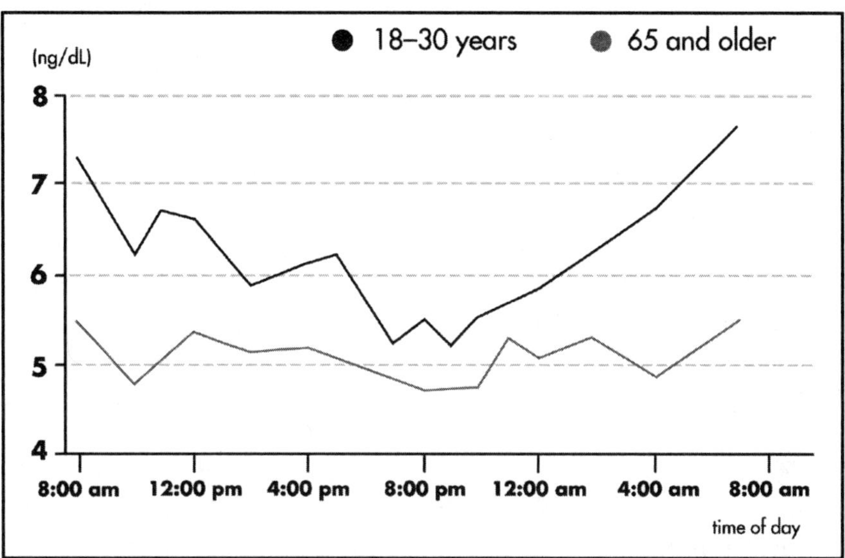

The daily testosterone production rhythm in younger and older men. (Note that the basic pattern is the same for both younger and older men, even though the amounts of testosterone are different.)

morning, and then builds up again throughout the day, finally beginning to drop off again in the evening. In fact, your morning "cup of T" is about 30% higher than it is when at its daily low point.

The Measure of a Man

Hormones are messengers, but who are the recipients of those messages? Not just anyone. If your postman delivered someone else's mail to your mailbox, you'd reject it, wouldn't you? Only mail addressed to you is allowed in your mailbox. It's the same thing with testosterone, and any other hormone. Your body's postman (the bloodstream) delivers testosterone to various mailboxes ("androgen receptors") along its route. These are the places in the body that are characteristically—even mythologically—associated with testosterone. Let's look at them in detail.

The Brain

Testosterone has a major influence over three important brain functions: cognitive function and memory, mood, and libido (sex drive). Let's take a look at each.

Cognitive Function and Memory. In a study conducted at Oregon Health & Science University[5], 30 men—16 healthy men, and 14 men undergoing "androgen deprivation treatment" for prostate cancer—were shown a list of words. Later, they were shown another list containing some of the words they'd just seen, as well as new words, and were asked which of the words they had already seen. The researchers found that while testosterone-deficient men were able to store items over the short term as well as non-deficient men, there was a sharp drop in retention after the two-minute mark. The researchers concluded that testosterone deprivation has a negative effect on the hippocampus, the part of the brain responsible for converting short-term memories into mid- or long-term.

Mood. Testosterone may play a role in keeping depression at bay. In a study of 278 men age 44 and older, those with a steep drop in testosterone levels (a condition known as hypogonadism, which we will discuss later) were 22% more likely to experience depression.[6]

Libido. The popular thinking is often that testosterone alone equals libido. No doubt about it, less testosterone often means diminished libido, and more testosterone leads to higher libido. But libido is really the product of a sort of team effort. Testosterone may be the captain of that team, but it's important to understand the concept holistically. It's much more complex than just free-floating levels of a single hormone. In fact, libido is linked to a number of factors, including (but not limited to) the following:

- Cardiovascular health
- Stress levels and overall mental health
- Sleep quality and quantity
- History of sexual abuse
- High alcohol consumption or use of controlled substances
- Diet and exercise patterns
- Infidelity
- Chronic conditions, including type 2 diabetes, hypothyroidism, or anemia

What's more, there's no way to measure libido objectively. (A report published in January, 2005[7] claims that an objective test that measures brainwaves is now available, but testing of this method is still in the early stages.) Rather, the best measure we have is subjective, usually involving a patient's answer to a questionnaire, and there is no single questionnaire accepted as the standard.

The Bones

During puberty, the overall growth in the height of the body starts at the skeletal level. The bones are equipped with androgen receptors, which allow them to interpret the signal necessary for growing, but also to continue the lifelong cycle of breakdown and renewal.

The Blood

Testosterone interacts with marrow in bone (and also kidneys) and helps produce red blood cells. However, there is such a thing as too much of a good thing. An overabundance of testosterone (which we sometimes see in athletes who abuse steroids, or patients overdosing on prescription testosterone) can lead to an abnormally high red blood cell count, a condition known as polycythemia. Testosterone is an anabolic substance, which means that it facilitates the creation of new tissue, including red blood cells.

The Prostate

Also at puberty, the presence of testosterone stimulates the growth and development of the prostate gland, the walnut-sized gland that surrounds the urethra, and is responsible for producing semen, the fluid that delivers sperm through ejaculation. The cells of the prostate are very responsive to a byproduct of testosterone, and as we'll discuss later on, that's a cause for concern for men who receive testosterone replacement therapy. Ironically, even as testosterone begins to decline with age (which we'll discuss at length soon), the prostate begins to grow again in about half of all men, a condition known as benign prostatic hyperplasia (or BPH for short). Despite much speculation, it's still not known exactly what causes BPH, but it is known that men who receive testosterone also notice increased prostate size, and its attendant symptoms, including frequent, weak, and nighttime urination, and in some cases, prostatic pain.

Synovial Tissue

Some researchers suggest a link between abnormal testosterone levels and rheumatoid arthritis, leading some to conclude that testosterone somehow acts directly on the synovium, the tissue that encases the joints. We'll discuss that later on, but for now, there's no scientific evidence that synovial tissue relies on testosterone for any of its function or integrity.

THE ARTERIES

It's equally unclear at the moment if testosterone has any effect on the endothelium, the cells that line the arterial tree, despite some working theories.

THE SEX ORGANS

At puberty, testosterone plays a key role in signaling the body to begin to let the testicles enlarge and descend, and for the penis to enlarge. But when puberty is complete (at around age 18 or so), the ride's over—which is a good news/bad news situation. More testosterone after puberty won't affect the size of the penis or testicles one way or another, but neither will less testosterone.

THE VOCAL CORDS

Also at puberty, testosterone acts on the vocal cords to make them larger and thicker, producing the characteristically manly deep voice. (Centuries ago, a rather gruesome—yet somewhat common—practice was to castrate young male choir singers so that their voices would never deepen.) Again, this is something of a one-shot deal. Once testosterone has done its work during puberty, it has relatively little effect after that. When testosterone begins naturally declining with age, the voice does not rise correspondingly, nor would extra testosterone help to deepen it.

FACIAL AND BODY HAIR

Another tell-tale mark of puberty is the development of facial and body hair. The follicles that produce that hair grow in response to testosterone. And again, a decline in testosterone doesn't necessarily correspond to a loss of facial or body hair. However, the follicles that were there since birth (the ones on the head) may end up being negatively affected by testosterone—at least indirectly—in some men. One of the byproducts of testosterone has a destructive effect on the hair follicles of the scalp in men who are genetically predisposed to baldness. That's not to say that bald men necessarily have higher testosterone (though many might like to think that they do!), but that the testosterone they do have is at least indirectly responsible for lack of hair on the scalp.

The Seminiferous Tubules

The testicles are essentially a coiled network of small tubes called seminiferous tubules, which are responsible primarily for producing sperm. Testosterone is part of the sperm-production process, but as I mentioned, it plays only a bit part. Luteinizing hormone (LH) is what's most important, and in fact an overabundance of testosterone can affect the brain in such a way as to diminish LH production. This partly explains why many athletes who abuse steroids become—at least temporarily—infertile.

The Skeletal Muscles

Your body has three basic kinds of muscle: cardiac muscle, which is found only in the heart; smooth muscle, such as that found in the digestive tract; and skeletal muscle, which you can voluntarily contract for bodily movement—or just flex in front of the mirror. At puberty, testosterone signals the body to increase its skeletal muscle mass, dramatically changing the composition of the body. For better or worse, muscle tissue remains responsive to testosterone throughout life. That means that a decrease in testosterone will typically also mean a decrease in muscle (along with an increase in fat), and that more testosterone means more muscle. That's why so many athletes, bodybuilders, and plain old image-

Turning Up the T

Not to cramp its style or anything, but when it comes to the sheer strength of androgen action, testosterone isn't the most potent hormone. No, that would be its close cousin dehydrotestosterone, or DHT for short. DHT action is a whopping five times more potent on androgen receptors, so those receptors use a chemical called 5-alpha reductase to convert testosterone to DHT. But don't worry; testosterone still deserves its reputation as head hormone in charge. It's just that it plays more of a managerial role, delegating multiple tasks to multiple "departments" of the body. It is the primary fuel with which the body powers its man-making machinery.

conscious civilians may be tempted to try boosting their testosterone, whether through prescribed medicine, illegal steroids, or any manner of supplements and other tactics.

But Will It Make a Guy Crush a Beer Can on His Head?

Is it really testosterone that makes some men act, as Phoebe would say, "testosteroney"? It's an important question to answer, because so-called "testosterone poisoning" has been blamed for certain acts of violence and aggression that are more common among males, including rape and murder.

But stepping up to the plate to defend testosterone is a bit of a no-win situation. We may be able to clear testosterone's good name, but at the end of the day, testosterone or no testosterone, we're still left with the fact that men are the more aggressive sex. However, because our topic here is testosterone, let's take a rational look at just how much of a part—if it plays one at all—the hormone plays in male behavior.

The problem with trying to single out testosterone is that behavior is such a delicate mingling of multiple factors that it's rather difficult to say what the precise effect of any of those factors is. There are genetic factors, social factors, environmental factors, psychological factors, and, let's not forget, *several other* hormonal factors aside from testosterone in the equation, and it's likely to be the interaction among all elements—something like a chemical reaction—that results in a given behavior. On the other hand, we see what happens when testosterone rises or falls. It's undeniable. When testosterone decreases, so does libido and, consequently, so do certain areas of sexual behavior. When testosterone is increased, a man's libido and (if he's lucky) frequency of sexual activity increases as well. Even taking a broader look at a man's personality, rather than an isolated view of one or two behaviors, one has only to watch your average pre-teen boy hit puberty. A tidal surge of testosterone, and all of a sudden, the kid becomes obnoxious. Adolescence is also the time of life when violent behavior is the most frequent and severe among males who commit violent acts.

Fanning the flames of this argument is something we just discussed: the brain has testosterone receptors, meaning that testosterone is at least partly involved in relaying messages that involve action and behavior. Further damning evidence is derived from a study conducted in the late

1980s. Researchers measured the testosterone of 89 male prison inmates and found that the inmates with higher testosterone concentrations had more often been convicted of violent crimes. In the housing unit, inmates rated as "tougher" by their peers also had higher testosterone.[8] Case closed, jury dismissed. It would seem pretty open-and-shut: Testosterone equals machismo, lunk-headedness, and aggressiveness.

But of course things are never quite that simple. Clearly, some relationship between testosterone and behavior exists. The question is: What is that relationship?

To start with, a later study of prison inmates showed that those with higher testosterone also had higher levels of cortisol, a steroid hormone produced by the adrenal cortex.[9] The researchers hypothesized that "Cortisol may be a biological indicator of psychological variables (e.g., social withdrawal) that moderate the testosterone-behavior relationship."

Another factor is that one of the symptoms of low testosterone happens to be irritability and anxiety—a dangerous cocktail. There may be equal valence to the claim that men with *low* testosterone are some of the grumpiest guys around, and just as likely as anyone—if not more so—to behave aggressively. Add to that the fact that while, yes, aggressive behavior *declines* along with declining testosterone, it doesn't stop altogether. Animal castration studies prove this phenomenon, where aggressiveness continues despite the animal have virtually zero testosterone. What's more, researchers have been able to reinstate aggressive behaviors in animals by replacing only a very small amount of testosterone, killing the theory that aggressiveness and testosterone are directly proportional. Robert Sapolsky, the famous Stanford University professor of biological sciences, explains it this way in his essay, "The Trouble with Testosterone":

> It's one of the more subtle points in endocrinology—what's referred to as a hormone having a "passive effect." Remove someone's testes and, as noted, the frequency of aggressive behavior is likely to plummet. Reinstate pre-castration levels of testosterone by injecting the hormone, and pre-castration levels of aggression typically return. Fair enough. Now, this time castrate an individual and restore testosterone levels to only 20 percent of normal. Amazingly, normal pre-castration levels of aggression come back.

> Castrate and now introduce twice the testosterone levels from before castration, and the same level of aggressive behavior returns. You need some testosterone around for normal aggressive behavior. Zero levels after castration, and down it usually goes; quadruple levels (the sort of range generated in weight lifters abusing anabolic steroids), and aggression typically increases. But anywhere from roughly 20 percent of normal to twice normal and it's all the same. The brain can't distinguish among the wide range of basically normal values.... Testosterone isn't causing aggression; it's exaggerating the aggression that's already there.

Another counterclaim: aggressive and violent behavior may be higher among men with higher testosterone, but that's a far cry from saying that all men with relatively high levels tend toward aggressiveness. Similarly, take a man with high levels of testosterone who is given to overly aggressive behavior, and watch him throughout the day. Because testosterone is highest in the morning, you'd assume that would be prime time for an aggressive act. In fact you could further infer that most violence in a society would be committed in the morning, as that's when the societal testosterone level is at its highest. And you'd be wrong on both counts.

Then there's what appears to be a chicken-or-the-egg effect. Is it too-high testosterone that leads to "male" behavior, or is it that certain behaviors (or exposure to certain stimuli) raise testosterone? Is behavior the *result* of hormone levels, or the *cause* of them? Research suggests that—at least some of the time—it's the latter. In one test researchers attended a college basketball game and asked male spectators if they'd like to participate in a study that measured their salivary testosterone before and after the game.[10] Of the eight men (ranging in age from 20 to 42 years), four supported the home team, and four supported the visiting team. The results showed that the fans who supported the winning team had a rise in testosterone shortly after the game, and fans of the losing team showed a drop. The rise shown in fans of the winners was large enough to reverse the normal decline in testosterone levels across the day. (It was a close game, and the final outcome wasn't predictable until the last seconds. The researchers concluded that this fact means that the rise in testosterone must have been sudden, rather than steady throughout the game.) In another, larger study, the same phenomenon resulted from men watching World Cup soccer on television. Still other studies have shown rises in testosterone after sex.

The bottom line appears to be that testosterone is a part of the behaviors we think of as decidedly male, but not the whole story.

The Low-Down

No question about it: testosterone is one manly hormone. It grunts, it groans, it hoards the remote control, and leaves the toilet seat up. And while it's shrouded in much mystery and mythology, we can say these things for sure:

- Testosterone is a steroid hormone that's largely responsible for developing the gender-specific characteristics of all males, both during fetal development and puberty.
- It is produced primarily in the testicles, with help from hormones produced in the brain, and a small amount of testosterone is produced by the adrenal glands.
- It is delivered through the bloodstream to the many androgen receptor sites of the body.
- Some receptor sites (such as the vocal cords) are significant only during puberty. Others (such as the bones, prostate, and skeletal muscles) remain responsive to the presence or lack of testosterone throughout your lifetime.
- Testosterone has an undeniable effect on behavior, but then again, so do several other things. But claims that testosterone equals aggression are myth.

CHAPTER 2:

ARE TESTOSTERONE LEVELS AN ISSUE FOR YOU?

YOU MAY HAVE PICKED UP THIS BOOK BECAUSE you're concerned that you—or someone you know—might have a problem with abnormal testosterone levels. This chapter will help you figure out how to tell if this is the case. As discussed in the last chapter, testosterone plays an important role in the body, and having just the right amount is an important part of being a healthy man or woman. In this chapter we'll take a look at some of the common symptoms associated with low testosterone, as well as symptoms of—yes, there is such a thing in some cases—too-high testosterone. We'll then examine how testosterone is measured, and what the results may mean for you.

Welcome to Adulthood—May I Take Your Testosterone?

Here's the part where I reveal the cold, hard truth. If you're in your early to mid-thirties, you almost definitely have less testosterone than you used to. It's one of nature's cruel little jokes: Just when you've escaped your freewheeling twenties with as many brain cells (and as few tattoos) as you could, and entered the age when you officially become an adult man, the very chemical essence of your manhood begins to slip away. It's true what they say: Youth is wasted on the young. As I mentioned in the last chapter, testosterone is present in the womb to help a male fetus develop properly, and then it remains largely dormant until puberty—

'round about age 12. During adolescence it is at its natural lifetime high and then levels off throughout the late teens and twenties. Starting at about age 30 (but it can be as late as 40 for some men) testosterone production begins to drop. From there on in, you'll continue to have less and less with each passing year, along with more gray hairs, wrinkles, and solicitations to join the AARP. It's called getting older, and—at least not yet—there's not much you can do about it. In chapter 1 we looked at several areas of the body that rely on testosterone to maintain their function or integrity. Some, like the vocal cords and sex organs, require testosterone only to ensure their proper development during puberty. Others, like the bones, muscles, and the brain, react to the presence, or lack, of testosterone throughout your life. To make a long story short, when testosterone declines, there are symptoms that go with it, and we'll discuss those symptoms below.

However, as we'll also discuss later, it's only when the symptoms of abnormal testosterone levels have an acute effect on quality of life that we begin to examine treatment options. The question of whether you have low testosterone all but answers itself: If you're 35 or older, you do. The question, then, is: Do you have abnormally, or dangerously, low testosterone?

How Much is Enough?

Remember the old saying, "a little dab'll do ya"? For all its potency, testosterone isn't produced in huge batches. In fact, its official unit of measurement is in nanograms (billionths of a gram) per deciliter (one tenth of a liter) of blood, expressed as ng/dL. That's barely a drop in the bucket. And as we'll discuss later on, most of what little testosterone you do produce never makes it to the body's receptor sites. Rather, it gets stuck to certain proteins in the blood that seem to want to keep testosterone all to themselves.

How much testosterone is enough? It's a bit of a tough question to answer. Remember from the last chapter that blood levels of testosterone rise and fall throughout the day, reaching their 24-hour peak in the early morning, before tapering off, and then inching back upward again in the early evening hours. Furthermore, as just mentioned, testosterone begins to drop off between age 30 and 40, and continues declining throughout life. In the end, assessing healthy levels of testosterone involves placing your levels on a spectrum. At the high end would be a young man under 30. We'll leave pubescent boys out of this discussion, because they're rarely checked for testosterone problems, barring evidence of some kind of injury or disease. (See the next chapter for more details.) At the other end—well, it's hard to say where to draw the line because testosterone declines continuously throughout life, and we're living longer and longer these days. Also, several other factors work in tandem with testosterone to determine whether there's any health risk involved. Furthermore, different spectra exist, depending on whom you ask. I'll split the difference here by taking the average values from each end of the spectrum: Healthy levels of testosterone are between 700 ng/dL and 1,100 ng/dL. Anything below 700 would be considered unhealthily low, and—while it's rare—anything above 1,100 would be considered unhealthily high.

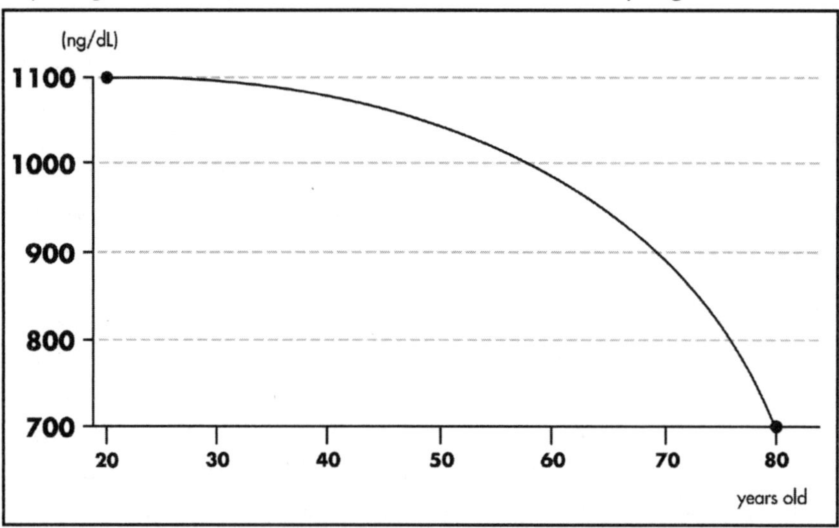

Average testosterone readings based on age group. Testosterone reaches its lifetime peak during adolescence, and levels off through the late teens and twenties. At around age 30, the body begins producing less, a trend that will continue throughout life.

The Best Things In Life Aren't Free

These readings refer to the total testosterone in your blood. However, only about 5% of it is usable. The rest is stuck to a protein called sex-hormone-binding globulin (or SHBG, for short), which is like a little magnet that attracts testosterone. While you may have, say, 900 ng/dL of total testosterone, about 855 ng/dL is likely to be bound to SHBG, meaning that the testosterone is not considered "bioavailable" or "free."

And as we'll discuss elsewhere, one of the ways to "raise" your testosterone is to lower your SHBG levels, which for some (though not all) men may be possible through diet (see chapter 9).

But let's not vilify SHBG. It actually does what it does for a good reason. First of all, testosterone that's bound to SHBG is in the hormonal equivalent of a minimum-security prison. The binding isn't terribly strong. Second, the SHBG isn't exactly taking testosterone away; it's storing it. Testosterone isn't very soluble in water (and thus, not in blood), so SHBG serves as a nice little reservoir for possible future use. The loosely bound testosterone becomes a readily available backup supply.

When Is It a Problem?

What's also important—*very important*—to understand is the difference between testosterone levels that are undesirably low, and those that are unhealthily low. The clinical term for unhealthily or dangerously low testosterone is "hypogonadism," and it is characterized by abnormally low testosterone, due to some kind of injury or disorder. Some genetic disorders, for instance, suppress normal production of testosterone. (Again, see chapter 3 for details.) Hypogonadism puts those who have it at a significant risk of bone fractures and possibly weight problems (which can lead to other health problems) due to the increase in body fat that accompanies abnormally low testosterone.

True hypogonadism is somewhat rare, and is almost never the result of normal, healthy aging. However, some people have begun to refer to the gradual decline in testosterone due to aging as Symptomatic Late-Onset Hypogonadism (SLOH). We'll learn more about this in chapter 5.

All normal, healthy men experience a decrease in testosterone, but are the effects more a quality-of-life issue than a health issue? We'll pick up that debate later on in this book, but for now, let's turn our attention to the common symptoms and occurrences that accompany a decline in testosterone levels.

We'll start out here with what's known as the ADAM (Androgen Deficiency in the Aging Male) questionnaire, developed by researchers at St. Louis University School of Medicine. While this survey is considered "highly predictive" of low testosterone, the symptoms mentioned may also be linked to several other health conditions, including depression, anxiety, physical exhaustion, and others. In other words, when it comes to diagnosing low testosterone, don't try this at home. On the other hand, many of the symptoms of testosterone deficiency are usually ignored at first, written off as the results of stress, poor diet, lack of excitement in life, or other intangibles. In most cases, it's the "softer" symptoms (i.e. those that can't be measured definitively) that are the first to appear in a testosterone-deficient man, followed by the more physically measurable ones.

The ADAM questionnaire asks about 10 specific symptoms:

1. Decrease in sex drive
2. Lack of energy
3. Decrease in strength and or endurance, or both
4. Lost height
5. Decreased "enjoyment of life"
6. Sadness or grumpiness, or both
7. Less strength in erections
8. Deterioration in sports ability
9. Falling asleep after dinner
10. Decreased work performance

If you feel that you are experiencing symptoms 1 or 7, or a combination of any 4 of the other symptoms on a long-term basis, you may have grounds to go to your doctor for more information about your testosterone levels, and possible treatments. However, it's important to keep in mind that the above symptoms serve as only a loose set of *guidelines* for assessing the likelihood of androgen deficiency and are not absolute criteria for androgen deficiency.

Furthermore, not everyone with testosterone deficiency will have these symptoms. They are based on the most basic and visible symptoms. Other common symptoms of low testosterone include the following:

Difficulty Concentrating and Forgetfulness. Scientists in the Oregon Health & Science University tested the ability of men undergoing testosterone deprivation therapy as part of prostate cancer treatment to remember words from a list, and compared the results to those for men who had normal levels of testosterone. The men were shown a list of words, and then, after two minutes, were shown another list that contained some of the words they had just seen as well as some new words. They were asked regarding each word on the list whether they had seen it before. The researchers found that for men undergoing the testosterone deprivation therapy, after two minutes there was a significant drop in the ability to remember the words. The researchers concluded that very low testosterone levels may affect a structure of the brain known as the hippocampus, which controls learning and memory.[11]

Altered Body Composition. Your body weight is more than just numbers on a scale—there's also body composition to consider. That is, the proportion of body fat to "lean mass"—the bone, muscle, and other non-fat materials of the body. Because testosterone is partly responsible for the building and maintenance of muscle bulk, as well as the metabolism that keeps your calorie-burning furnace fired up throughout the day, a deficiency may tip the compositional balance in favor of body fat. That means that your overall body weight may not change much, but the fat-to-lean mass ratio will. This can result in a decrease in physical strength, as well as what's referred to as a "female fat distribution," in which fat is deposited in the midsection in a way that is more consistent with a normal female body (notably, pronounced deposits around the hips and breasts) than a male body.

Decrease in Typical Male Hair Patterns and Locations. As we discussed in chapter 1, testosterone is responsible for several "secondary" sexual characteristics, including body and facial hair. A lack of body or facial hair doesn't necessarily mean problems with testosterone levels. Some men are naturally more hairy than others. However, a *sudden* and *dramatic* thinning of your facial or body hair may in some cases suggest testosterone depletion, and most men will notice a gradual thinning, becoming more pronounced in later years.

Decreased Bone Density. In severe cases of testosterone depletion in men, as in cases when the testicles are surgically removed—which occurs in some treatment programs for prostate cancer, or in the case of male-to-female transsexuals—bone density drops to dangerously low levels and puts the person at almost certain risk of developing osteoporosis unless treatment is given. This, however, is rarely a concern for the average man undergoing gradual declines in testosterone as a result of normal aging. However, some bone loss can be expected for almost any man due to the gradual decrease that comes with age. Question 4 of the ADAM questionnaire asks about lost height for just that reason. As bone material from the spine becomes weaker and more porous, a stooping posture often becomes more pronounced, producing a decrease in stature.

Depression. Depression and testosterone levels can be a bit of a chicken-or-egg problem. As we'll discuss in the next chapter, depression itself may be a factor in lowering testosterone levels in an otherwise young, healthy male. Likewise, depression could be a symptom of testosterone depletion. In other cases, the physical symptoms of low testosterone —including low energy, low sex drive, and difficulty concentrating— may mimic the symptoms of depression, without having all of the characteristics of this psychological disorder.

Low Fertility. As testosterone plays a role in sperm development, lower testosterone may lead to lowered sperm count significant enough to affect fertility levels. As we discussed in the last chapter, testosterone is produced in the testes' Leydig cells. The testes also produce sperm in the seminiferous tubules, but only when sufficient testosterone levels are present. In the case of the normally aging man, though, this is not a major cause for concern. The testes do have a higher concentration of testosterone than other body parts do in order to facilitate this sperm production. Apparently, not much testosterone, relatively speaking, is required for sperm production (a subtle drop in sperm production is a normal part of aging). That may be part of the reason why a normal 70-year-old man may have only about half the testosterone he did as a teenager, but is still often able to father children.

Decrease in Energy. Testosterone is part of the body's system that produces red blood cells. As a result, a sharp drop-off in testosterone levels can lead to a corresponding drop-off in red blood cells, producing anemia, the symptoms of which include low energy, exhaustion, and chronic tiredness. A decrease in energy may also result from the decreased muscle mass and increased fat levels that often accompany testosterone deficiency, which has a profound effect on metabolism.

Erectile Dysfunction. While we know that testosterone has a significant effect on sex drive and overall sexual function, you may be surprised to find out that lowered testosterone is not a frequent cause of erectile dysfunction. Referring back to chapter 1, we see that testosterone plays a role in erectile function in something of a behind-the-scenes manner. It has more to do with interest and desire, which in turn sets in motion the physical processes resulting in erection. But, as I'll mention several times throughout this book, erectile dysfunction is often the result of a combination of varying degrees of physical, mental, and emotional issues working together.

Too Much Testosterone

Generally speaking, as far as most men are concerned, the more testosterone they have, the better. High testosterone levels are rarely something to complain about. Unless, that is, you have prostate cancer. Earlier we learned about a study conducted on men who were receiving testosterone deprivation therapy as part of a prostate-cancer treatment program. Testosterone deprivation, known as "ablation," is normally conducted through a surgical removal of the testicles, or through administering medicines that block production of testosterone and other hormones. This is because there appears to be a link between lowered levels of testosterone and higher levels of T-lymphocytes ("T cells"), the white blood cells that can fight against tumor cells and infections. (T cells are also thought to help other immune cells known as "B cells" make antibodies to defend the body against certain bacterial and fungal infections, and possibly against cancer.) Researchers at the Mayo Clinic, conducting testosterone-depletion experiments on mice, found that the presence of testosterone slows or weakens the response of T cells and that that without testosterone, T cells "turn-on" more quickly.[12]

Too much testosterone has also been associated with a decrease in luteinizing hormone, and thus a decrease in fertility. However, such too-high levels almost never occur naturally, and are almost always the result of abusing artificial testosterone (see chapters 6 and 7).

Getting Your Testosterone Measured

If you're concerned about your testosterone levels, it's time to talk to your doctor. Measuring testosterone, and diagnosing low testosterone, is less intimidating than you may think.

As we mentioned earlier, the symptoms of testosterone depletion are often similar to those of other conditions, including stress, depression, or exhaustion, or even more serious conditions. (Also, as we'll discuss in the next chapter, some serious health conditions, including diabetes, often

A Word About Home Testing

IT TAKES ONLY A FEW MOMENTS ON THE INTERNET to discover many manufacturers offering home testosterone testing kits. These kits normally cost about $65 and require you to provide a saliva sample that is mailed to a lab operated by the manufacturer. (Interestingly, some states have laws prohibiting such tests.) While there's no direct evidence to say that mail-order medical tests are better or worse than a more conventional blood test method, tests that use a cotton dental roll to collect a saliva sample often lead to inflated testosterone scores. (Believe it or not, sugar-free gum seems to work better as a collection material.)[13]

Then there's always the question of "why?" Mail-order tests claim to be 100% confidential, so there might be an appeal if you happen to be especially timid, for whatever reason, about discussing testosterone talking with your doctor. But these tests cannot provide the kind of personalized analysis and care—and cross-referencing of test results with your existing medical records—as can a test performed by your doctor.

That said, a home test may, in a way similar to home pregnancy testing kits, provide you a springboard for a conversation with your doctor. A man concerned about his testosterone would likely want to check his levels because he's experienced some or all of the symptoms described earlier in this chapter. The bottom line is that home testing is harmless, but no substitute for a thorough exam with your doctor.

also contribute to low testosterone.) Likewise, you may go to your doctor complaining of sexual difficulties, or difficulty concentrating, only to be told that you are experiencing depression or anxiety. While it is important to rule out all other underlying conditions, when talking to your doctor, make certain to frame the conversation in a way that includes your concern about your testosterone levels. The standard thinking today is that only men who are experiencing symptoms should be evaluated.

Testing, Testing...

You may bring the question of testosterone levels to your primary care physician, or ask to be referred to a urologist or endocrinologist. Either way, your doctor may likely begin the process by conducting the ADAM questionnaire discussed earlier, or something similar. After all, if none of the symptoms from the ADAM questionnaire is present, there's little need to explore further the possibility of testosterone deficiency, and your doctor will likely consider other underlying causes of your symptoms.

If, however, your doctor believes that your answers to the questionnaire are enough to warrant further exploration, he or she will likely conduct a routine physical examination, and then a more specific exam that addresses many of the symptoms and effects of significant testosterone deficiency that we've discussed throughout this chapter, including changes in muscle strength, body composition, body and facial hair, and posture. If you are over age 45, your doctor will likely also conduct a prostate examination, including a test for prostate-specific antigens, which are a fairly reliable indicator of possible prostate cancer or infection or inflammation of the gland.

Again—and with the exception of the prostate exam—the examination up to this point is based on subjective data, and many men are tempted to determine for themselves one way or the other whether they have a problem with testosterone levels and whether they should do anything about it. But your doctor is also able to conduct highly specific laboratory tests, including blood levels of testosterone, blood levels of pituitary hormones (to determine if the possible deficiency is linked to an abnormality of the pituitary gland), and in some cases, a bone-density scan (to check for osteoporosis), and semen-level tests of the ejaculate.

Your blood test will likely be conducted in the morning because that's when your body's levels are at their peak of their daily production cycles. A reading below 200 ng/dL may be cause for a follow-up exam to see if your testosterone is consistently low, or if it was temporarily suppressed by any of the contributing factors we'll discuss in the next chapter. This reading refers to total, and not "free," testosterone, however.

Measuring free testosterone is a bit of a sticky subject, and not everyone agrees on the best method to truly assess a baseline of free levels. Different labs have their own methods. And because even 1 ng/dL can make a real difference one way or the other, it's easy to see how this can become controversial. As a general rule, an average healthy man uses only roughly 5% of his total testosterone, depending on SHBG levels so multiplying your total testosterone by 0.05 will yield a fairly safe ballpark figure.

The Low-Down

Testosterone is related to several areas of physical, mental, and emotional well-being, and so extreme fluctuations of testosterone levels can have adverse health effects, or at least undesirable symptoms. Here's the low-down on testosterone levels:

- Levels considered normal are between 300 and 1,000 ng/dL of blood. This spectrum factors in fluctuating levels throughout the day, and declining levels over the average lifespan.
- "Total testosterone" represents the amount of the hormone found in the blood, expressed in ng/dL. However, the vast majority of it is bound to blood proteins that keep it from being delivered to the body's androgen receptors. It is the "free" or "bioavailable" testosterone that matters most when we discuss symptoms of testosterone-level issues.
- There are several symptoms associated with low testosterone levels, but which are also associated with other common health issues. There is a difference between testosterone that is undesirably low, and testosterone that is dangerously low.
- High testosterone is rarely a significant health issue, unless it coincides with some other health problem or is caused by abuse of artificial testosterone.
- The only way to know if your testosterone is low is to receive a medical test, preferably during the early-morning hours.

CHAPTER 3:

WHAT AFFECTS TESTOSTERONE LEVELS?

SO FAR WE'VE TAKEN A LOOK AT WHAT TESTOSTERONE is and does, how it is produced, and the effects on the body and mind when levels drop below their desired and healthy range. In this chapter we'll explore many of the common—and not so common—ways in which testosterone levels are raised or lowered, whether temporarily or permanently.

As I've mentioned in the previous two chapters, every man who is 35 years or older has less testosterone than he did as an adolescent, and will have less and less with each passing year for the remainder of his life. Aging, then, is by far the most common—but least dramatic—cause of falling testosterone levels, affecting a full 100% of the male human race. Again, beginning somewhere in his early to mid thirties, a healthy man will begin to decrease testosterone production by about one percent per year, with the physical and mental effects becoming noticeable by about age 45 or so. Even so, by age 45 (sometimes considered the beginning of "middle age") the man has noticed only a 10% drop in his testosterone—nothing to sneeze at, but nothing earth-shattering either.

It's not just a decline in overall production that leads to the noticeable effects of decreasing testosterone. Instead, it's a one-two punch. Not only does the body produce less testosterone, but it produces more of the villainous sex-hormone-binding globulin (SHBG) that we discussed in chapter 2. That means that the diminishing supply of testosterone that is produced becomes increasingly less "bioavailable" or "free."

But let's get back to this idea of normal testosterone declines and their effects on an otherwise healthy aging man. At an average 10% drop per decade, a healthy man of 70 years is likely to have seen only a 40% drop from his peak testosterone productions—a bit more dramatic, yes, but still not enough of a drop to altogether halt sperm production, sexual function, libido, facial-hair growth, and other male characteristics.

Understanding this begins to answer the question of whether there is truly such a thing as "male menopause," also referred to as andropause, which we'll discuss in greater detail in chapter 4. It seems like almost every week the media is touting some story about a 75-year-old man (usually a famous actor or business man, with a 20-something wife) fathering a child. Actor Tony Randall became a first-time father at age 77!

However, in addition to the normal, one-percent yearly decline, there are several other conditions under which testosterone fall-off can be dramatically accelerated to the point of causing not only undesirable mind-and-body effects (as in low sex drive, diminished mood), but also posing significant health risks, including osteoporosis, severely weakened musculature, and anemia.

Let's start with the most radical of these conditions: removal of the testicles. As we discussed in chapter 1, for a man, about 95% of his testosterone is produced by his testicles, the other five percent is produced by the adrenals. Remove a testicle (as happens in cases of testicular cancer, the most common form of cancer for men in their 20s), and you'll decrease testosterone by about 45%. Remove both testicles (as happens in some men undergoing treatment for prostate cancer, or male-to-female transsexuals) and you've all but wiped out testosterone from the body.

But of course not all causes have such an extreme effect. As for those other causes, I've broken them down into the following broad categories:

1. Genetic and developmental factors
2. Injury, disease, or disease treatment
3. Environmental, social, and lifestyle factors

Let's take a look at each in greater detail.

Genetic and Developmental Factors

Sometimes low testosterone is destined from birth, or not long after, perhaps due to low exposure to testosterone in the womb (via the mother's placenta), which in turn inhibits full development of the male testosterone-producing machinery, through chromosomal disorders or other diseases that will affect testosterone production starting in adolescence, or through difficulties in proper course of puberty.

Klinefelter Syndrome

Chromosomally speaking, men have an X and a Y sex chromosome (women have two X chromosomes), but about one in 1,000 men is believed to have an extra copy of his X chromosome—a condition known as Klinefelter Syndrome. The syndrome often leads to impaired testosterone production beginning in puberty, and those who have it often have difficulty with fertility, due to smaller testicles that were not fully developed, and hence, less capable of producing adequate levels of sperm. (Low testosterone starting at this early age can also—but doesn't always—lead to female-style breast growth, known as gynecomastia, and reduced facial and body hair.) Because any chromosomal traits are passed down, Klinefelter Syndrome is, technically speaking, hereditary. But it is not a frequently inherited common trait like, say, blue eyes or blond hair (See John's story in chapter 6.)

Hereditary Hemochromatosis

One of the most common genetic disorders, hereditary hemochromatosis (iron overload) affects nearly two million Americans. The disorder is characterized by an abnormal absorption of iron.

Cryptorchidism

In the male fetus, the testicles begin their lives in the abdomen and from there, gradually grow in size and descend through the abdomen on their way to the their final home: the scrotum. In most boys, the testicles have reached the scrotum by birth; in others (6% to 10%) the testicles will descend in the first year after birth. However, for about one boy in 100, the testicles remain undescended, a condition known as cryptorchidism. Cryptorchid testicles are often corrected surgically within the first year of birth. When testicles are not brought to the scrotum by at least age four, the child is at risk of insufficient testosterone production (and thus, impaired development of primary and secondary sex characteristics) in adolescent and adult years.

Injury, Disease, or Disease Treatment

A number of illnesses are known to contribute to impaired testosterone production. Further, treatments for some diseases (that may or may not themselves cause lowered testosterone levels) lead to either temporary or permanent decline or outright cessation of normal testosterone production. Removal of the testicles, as mentioned earlier, is just the most dramatic example. Let's begin by looking at some diseases that affect testosterone.

DISEASES OF, OR TRAUMA TO, THE HYPOTHALAMUS OR PITUITARY GLAND

Remember from chapter 1 that while the testicles do the legwork in testosterone production, they cannot do so without the green light—in the form of chemical messengers—from the brain, particularly the hypothalamus, which produces GnRH, which in turn signals the pituitary gland to produce LH, which will travel to the testicles, signaling them to produce testosterone. When you are ill, your body produces less LH. Pituitary tumors lead to an increase in a chemical called prolactin, which in turn causes a decrease in sex hormone levels. Simply put, when these two structures of the brain don't work properly, whether due to head trauma or benign or cancerous tumors, neither does testosterone production.

INJURY OR TUMOR ON THE TESTICLES

In order to produce sperm, the testicles must live in the relatively cool climate of the scrotum. That's an advantage as far as fertility is concerned, but a disadvantage—as just about any man will tell you from all too painful experience—when it comes to the protection of these ever-so-sensitive organs. Because the scrotum has no bone or cartilage to protect its precious cargo, the testicles are especially prone to injury. Any manner of sports injury, violence, or unfortunate accident may be sufficient to cause temporary or permanent damage to one or both testicles, and in extreme cases, requiring surgical repair or removal of one or both testicles.

Inside the scrotum, the testicles are secured and suspended by structures known as spermatic cords, which sometimes get tangled, cutting off the supply of blood and nutrients to the organs. This results in pain, swelling, and tenderness. This so-called testicular torsion usually happens to younger men as a result of vigorous activity, but can also happen for no apparent reason. In either case, it is an acute event, requiring emergency care. If care is not given properly and immediately, permanent damage to the testicles can result.

The final problem that directly affects the testicles is a tumor on one or both. As mentioned earlier, this is among the most common of cancers in younger men. It is, however, in itself a rare form of cancer, characterized by a rapid and uncontrolled division of the cells of one or both testicles. The tumor or tumors may produce a lump on, or overall enlargement of, the testicles, or an unusual heaviness in the scrotum. Caught in time, and treated correctly, testicular cancer has a better than 90% cure rate, but often involves removal of one or both testicles (and sometimes some of the lymph nodes in the abdomen), and may also require chemotherapy or radiation treatment.

Sarcoidosis

Sarcoidosis is an inflammatory disease affecting the body's tissues. The inflammation is unique in that it produces small lumps (also called nodules or granulomas) in the tissues. One of the tissue sites that can be affected is that of the testicles, negatively affects testosterone production. This disease is relatively uncommon, affecting about 20 out of 100,000 people in America.

Diabetes

Type 2 diabetes (or adult onset diabetes) is the form of the disease in which the body becomes resistant to insulin, the hormone that transports sugars from the blood into the body's cells. Until 2004 it wasn't widely suspected that the disease may affect testosterone, but a large study from the State University of New York at Buffalo found hypogonadism in nearly one-third of 100 type-2 diabetics.[14]

It's still not clear exactly why or how diabetes acts on the body's testosterone-producing factory, but the hypogonadal men from this study also had lower levels of both luteinizing hormone and follicle-stimulating hormone, the two brain chemicals that work in conjunction with the testicles to produce testosterone. This finding suggests that type 2 diabetes likely acts on the pituitary or the hypothalamus, and not the testicles, to affect testosterone production.

HYPERTENSION

It's not known exactly why high blood pressure (hypertension) affects testosterone, but we know that it does simply because most men with hypertension also have lower testosterone. (Most men with hypertension are also over the age of 30, in which case they'd have lower testosterone anyway, so the precise magnitude of the effect of hypertension on testosterone may not always be crystal clear.) A major study of more than 1,100 men age 30 to 70 found that those who had hypertension (officially categorized a 160/95 or higher) had significantly lower testosterone levels than non-hypertensives, and that the higher the blood pressure, the lower the testosterone.

If that's not bad enough, chew on this: Hypertension is in almost every typical American's future—not because it's biologically predestined, but because of our infamous eating and exercise habits. If you're an American adult there is an almost one-in-three chance that you too have hypertension. It's estimated that 96 million Americans have the disease, which operates with such assassin-like stealth that it's been nicknamed "the silent killer." It has no symptoms, but nevertheless triples your risk of dying of a heart attack and increases the risk of a stroke sevenfold over people with normal blood pressure.The good news is that hypertension is preventable or manageable through diet and exercise (see chapters 8 and 9 for more.)

KIDNEY DISEASE

End-stage renal disease (a.k.a, renal failure) is a complete or near complete failure of the kidneys to perform their function of excreting wastes, concentrating urine, and regulating levels of the minerals in the blood that carry bioelectrical signals.

End-stage renal failure is associated with the increased production of a pituitary hormone called prolactin which, in too-high amounts, interferes with testosterone production. (However, end-stage renal failure is not thought to be the primary mechanism for the increase in prolactin. It's just that the two are usually found together.)

TREATMENT FOR PROSTATE CANCER

You might recall from a previous chapter that testosterone contributes to the acceleration of prostate cancer and that one possible treatment method is to take measures to lower testosterone in the body. It seems unnecessary to point out that testosterone-lowering medical treatments will lower your testosterone, but for the record, there are a couple of ways to go about it.

Hormone therapies are currently the main way to treat advanced prostate cancer, and most men with prostate cancer prefer it to surgical means (i.e., surgical castration). The three primary hormonal treatments are as follows:

1. **Luteinizing hormone-releasing hormone analogs** These drugs work by decreasing testosterone production to very low levels. LHRH analogs are administered via injection or small implants placed under the skin. One of the strange effects, though, is that prior to lowering testosterone, they cause a temporary spike in testosterone, something known as "tumor flare"). That's because these drugs are synthetic analogs of the luteinizing hormone-releasing hormone that stimulates production of luteinizing hormone, which in turn stimulates testosterone production. So during the first days of treatment, a patient's testosterone level will usually *rise* instead of falling, and that increase can stimulate briefly increased growth of prostate and prostate cancer cells. The response is transient in most patients, lasting for perhaps seven to ten days.
2. **Luteinizing hormone-releasing hormone antagonists** These drugs have recently been approved for use as hormone therapy in patients with advanced prostate cancer. LHRH antagonists lower testosterone levels more quickly than LHRH analogs, and don't cause tumor flare. On the other hand they carry a risk of serious and potentially life-threatening allergic reactions.
3. **Antiandrogens** These drugs work by blocking the effect of testosterone in the body. These drugs are sometimes used in addition to surgical castration in cases of highly advanced cancer.

Environmental, Social, and Lifestyle Factors

Sometimes it's factors outside the body that, when taken in through the five senses, lead to a temporary or more or less permanent decrease of testosterone production, to varying degrees. Some of them may surprise you. Of all the things that determine how much, or how little, testosterone your body produces, the following lifestyle factors are the most receptive to modification, and thus hold the most potential to affect your body's natural production of testosterone. We haven't yet touched on testosterone replacement therapy, but will in much detail in later chapters. For now, let's talk about *natural* production. You may not be able to control the fact that you are aging, and you may not always be able to control the genetic factors that may predispose you to any of the illnesses we've discussed in this chapter. And even the most cautious among us is sometimes prone to any of the accidents and injuries that might affect testosterone production.

But anybody willing to take the time, and develop the discipline, can control some or all of the lifestyle factors that may make an impact on testosterone. The following serves as a preview of upcoming chapters—namely 8 and 9—but for now, let's take the 30,000-foot view.

Stress

Our body's instinctual response to stressful situations—racing heart, clenched jaw, sweaty palms—is the classic fight-or-flight response that's been hard-coded into the human nervous system since the beginning of mankind. The physiological processes are priming your body with energy and muscle tension to either stand to face the enemy, or to run like hell. Back in your ancestors' days, stress meant staring down a hungry saber tooth tiger. Nowadays it means taking heat from the boss or braving rush-hour traffic. Problem is, your nervous system doesn't know the difference. The stress response is classified as a "non-specific" response, meaning it's a sort of one-size-fits-all approach to any situation that presents any level of perceived threat to your physical, mental, or emotional safety or well-being. (Compare that to a specific response like hunger, which happens if—and only if—you've been without food for too long.) Excessive stress is associated with increased production of the stress hormone cortisol, which suppresses testosterone production.

Excess stress also accelerates the aging process. One large study from Denmark[15] examined 431 men, all of whom were 51 years old. The researchers found that subjects with low levels of free testosterone, or those in the lowest quintile of the distribution of the hypogonadal index "showed a cluster of negative psychosocial variables, and psychological...problems." Those findings lead the researchers to conclude that "psychosocial stress may be associated with a process of premature ageing in middle-aged males, corresponding to a hypogonadal state."

Smoking

It's somewhat inconclusive how cigarette smoking affects testosterone. Some studies have suggested that it actually spurs an increase in luteinizing hormone levels from the pituitary, which in turn stimulated *increased* testosterone production from the testicles. On the other hand, smoking also seems to promote increased production of sex-hormone-binding globulin, which attaches to testosterone, holding it prisoner in the blood stream.

Smoking is also linked to high blood pressure (hypertension), which in turn has a negative effect on testosterone. One thing that's more certain: Whether or not it directly affects testosterone, smoking does increase your chances of developing a condition that's also associated with low testosterone: erectile dysfunction. After age 30, regular smokers increase their risk of erectile dysfunction by nearly 50%.

Testosterone or no testosterone, if you smoke, please try to quit. And if you're having trouble quitting, get help from your doctor.

Obesity

Sadly, in 2005, the number of Americans who will die of health complications related to excess bodyweight will be about equal to the number of children who will die in Ethiopia and Eritrea due to lack of food. Overweight and obesity have reached near epidemic proportions in our country, increasing threefold over the last three decades. Today, nearly two-thirds of Americans are considered overweight, and nearly one-third of them are considered obese.

Obesity is defined as a body mass index (a number representing one's proportion of height to weight) of 30 or more. Body mass indexes of 35 or higher are considered morbidly obese. (See chapter 9 to determine your own body mass index.)

How all this relates to testosterone is a bit hard to say exactly. Obesity contributes to the development of other health conditions that are known to lower testosterone, including hypertension and diabetes. Also, most people who are obese likely became obese by following a diet that contributes to increased production of SHBG, thereby lowering the availability of whatever testosterone they do produce, and decreased production of luteinizing hormone, which is essential for testosterone production. High concentrations of body fat are also related to what's known as aromatase activity, a process where testosterone is converted to estrogen. Body fat contains aromatase, so there is a proportional relationship between fat content and estrogen levels.

A major study[16] of more than 1,500 men found that those with a waist circumference of 102 cm (about 40 inches) had the lowest testosterone, despite age.

Diet

You might remember from the beginning of this chapter that as men age, not only does testosterone production decrease, but transport proteins (particularly SHBG) increase. These proteins bind to testosterone, making it unavailable to be used by the body's receptor sites. Adding to the problem is the fact that a diet low in protein has been shown to increase SHBG, thereby decreasing bioavailable testosterone. Researchers at the University of Massachusetts Medical School and the New England Research Institutes looked at 1,552 men with an average age of 55 who had filled out a diet and lifestyle questionnaire and from whom blood samples were taken to measure, among other things, testosterone levels. The researchers found an inverse relationship between protein and fiber, and SHBG levels. That is, men who ate diets higher in protein and fiber had less SHBG, and thus more bioavailable testosterone.[17] In chapter 9 we'll take a closer look at how diet affects testosterone levels, and how you can modify your diet to increase testosterone production, or at least increase the amount of bioavailable testosterone.

Alcohol Abuse

We'll cover this in more detail in chapter 9, but excess alcohol use is consistent with decreased testosterone levels because of the rather toxic effect it has on the body, which leads to atrophy (shrinkage) of the testes, reduction in follicle stimulating hormone and luteinzing hormone production, and increased cortisol production. Excessive consumption of "empty calories" leads to increased body fat, which in turn leads to increase aromatase activity, as described above. Excess alcohol use is also a major contributor to cirrhosis of the liver, which affects testosterone in turn. One of the liver's jobs is to metabolize estrogen, which all men produce in small amounts. But when the liver is cirrhotic, that metabolism doesn't happen, leading to a buildup in the blood, in turn contributing to further testicular atrophy, female-style breast growth, and other undesirable symptoms and traits.

Excessive exercise

Marathoners and long-distance cyclists may subject themselves to such grueling feats in part to show of their manliness, but endurance athletes typically have lower total testosterone than sedentary men of the same age. Why this is true is still a matter of debate, but one working theory is discussed in chapter 8.

Marriage or committed relationship

No need to backtrack—you read it right the first time. Researchers at Harvard decided to test whether a man's relationship status could be a meaningful predictor of testosterone levels. In one study, 122 male students of Harvard Business School provided saliva samples from which testosterone levels were tested, and also filled out a questionnaire having to do with his romantic relationship—or lack thereof. The results revealed that men in committed romantic relationships, including marriage, had 21% less testosterone than those who were not in such a relationship.[18] (Between those who were married and those who were in a committed relationship, there was no significant difference in testosterone levels.) The researchers concluded that such findings made evolutionary sense, as the lowered testosterone may play a part in lowering the man's libido just enough to make him more inclined to stay with the family than go out chasing other women. Other studies have shown testosterone to drop considerably just from holding a baby—or even a doll. There are no studies thus far to suggest that fatherhood by itself would lead to a drop in testosterone. But because this study mentions an evolutionary component, it doesn't seem to be much of a leap to infer that fatherhood is the desired result of a committed relationship. In other words, there may be a spectrum of testosterone loss, ranging from the beginning of a committed relationship and ending in fatherhood.

The Low-Down

Testosterone lowers with age, but age isn't the only factor associated with lower testosterone. Several other factors may work against you, depending on your genes, your lifestyle, and your medical history. The things that can also negatively affect your testosterone levels can be broken down as follows:

- Genetic and developmental factors, including Klinefelter Syndrome, hereditary hemochromatosis, and cryptorchidism.
- Injury, disease, or disease treatment, including diseases of the hypothalamus or pituitary gland, injury to the testicles, sarcoidosis, diabetes, hypertension, kidney disease, and treatment for prostate cancer.
- Environmental, social, and lifestyle factors, including stress, smoking, obesity, diet, alcohol abuse, excessive exercise, and marriage.

CHAPTER 4:

HEALTH PROBLEMS LINKED TO TESTOSTERONE LEVELS

IN CHAPTER 3 WE LOOKED AT HOW TESTOSTERONE can be negatively affected by certain diseases. Now we're going to look at some diseases that may in turn be *the result of* abnormal testosterone levels. We know that as age increases, so does the risk of certain serious diseases. At the same time, as age increases, testosterone *decreases*. Coincidence? Maybe, maybe not. In this short chapter we'll look at some of the latest research that compares testosterone levels with the prevalence of many common, but serious diseases, some specifically age-related, others not. Furthermore, while most of what we'll discuss below is linked to *low* testosterone, high testosterone can be a factor as well, as we'll see.

Alzheimer's Disease

Like bone, muscle, and skin, brain tissue is responsive to testosterone. Researchers have long wondered what that relationship between testosterone and the brain means for men whose testosterone levels drop as they age, especially as it relates to certain age-related brain disorders. Researchers have also wondered whether testosterone depletion contributes to, or results from, some disease processes.

In a letter to the Journal of the American Medical Association, researchers from the University of Southern California announced their findings that brain levels of testosterone are significantly lower in subjects with Alzheimer's disease compared with those who don't have the disease. They also found that brain levels of testosterone are also significantly reduced in men with mild neuropathology consistent with early-stage Alzheimer's.

As for that chicken-or-the-egg question of whether low testosterone depletion contributes to, or results from the disease, the USC researchers found that "testosterone depletion likely precedes, and thus may contribute to, rather than result, from the development of [Alzheimer's], since low brain testosterone is observed in men with early indications of [Alzheimer's] neuropathology."[19]

Depression

As we've discussed several times already, many of the symptoms of low testosterone mirror the common symptoms of depression, including lack of energy, low interest in sex, change of eating habits, and loss of interest in enjoyable activities. Doctors often make an initial diagnosis of depression before getting to the real root of the problem. What we haven't discussed yet is whether the two might be related. That is, whether low testosterone can not only produce depression-like symptoms, but actually increase the likelihood of depressive illness.

Researchers from the Veterans Affairs Puget Sound Health Care System in Seattle examined over a two-year period the medical records of 278 men age 45 years and older, who had no prior diagnosis of depressive illness, but who did have consistently normal or low testosterone. They found that during the two-year period, the men with low testosterone were three times more likely (21.7%, compared to 7.1%) to be diagnosed with clinical depression.[20]

Heart Disease

Because men have significantly more testosterone than women do, and also have a higher prevalence of heart disease, researchers have long thought that more testosterone equaled a higher risk of heart problems. Now, it looks like the very opposite might be true. Coronary Artery Disease (CAD) may be linked to low testosterone both directly and indirectly. First, as men age and testosterone naturally drops, body fat tends to increase. This increase is the result of a number of factors. Lower testosterone does typically lead to changed body composition, where body fat increases and muscle mass decreases. The increased body fat may also be compounded by an age-related slowing of the metabolism coupled with a decrease in physical activity. In chapters 8 and 9 we'll talk about how you can stabilize and even reverse some of these effects through diet and exercise, but for our purposes here, it's important to know that too much body fat is a known CAD risk factor. Researchers from the Charles R. Drew University of Medicine and Science in Los Angeles examined whether low testosterone might have a direct effect on the heart and arteries.

In a review of medical studies, there was no clear link between testosterone levels that rise or fall within the normal range. But in a series of animal studies, the researchers looked at how the presence of testosterone affects the development of hardened arteries, a condition known as artherosclerosis. The presence of testosterone was found to slow the onset of artherosclerosis. According to the researchers, "Testosterone concentrations either above or below the physiologic male range may increase the risk of atherosclerotic heart disease."[21]

Rheumatoid Arthritis

Clinicians have known for a long time that testosterone levels are low in people with rheumatoid arthritis, a type of chronic arthritis that occurs in joints on both sides of the body, such as hands or knees. (Rheumatoid arthritis is also known in some cases to affect the skin, eyes, lungs, heart, blood, nerves or kidneys.) Researchers have long wondered whether rheumatoid arthritis causes low testosterone, whether treatment for the condition may lower testosterone levels, or whether it's the low testosterone that leads to rheumatoid arthritis to begin with.

British scientist William James made the case that low testosterone could be a contributor to rheumatoid arthritis in a letter published in the Annals of Rheumatic Disease, where he cited cases of testosterone therapy improving arthritic symptoms. Further, he cited that rheumatoid arthritis is associated with the presence of certain immune-related molecules, which are themselves associated with low testosterone in men.[22]

The Low-Down

Low or high testosterone levels don't necessarily predict impending doom. However, if your levels have been found to be too low or too high, you'll likely want to keep a dialogue going with your doctor to monitor for some of the diseases we've mentioned here. It goes without saying that you'll want to discuss any family history of the above diseases, as well as any symptoms you may be experiencing. The low-down on disease and testosterone is this:

- Like diet, exercise, and genetic predisposition (among several other factors) testosterone too has an effect on your risk level of certain diseases.
- Testosterone levels may be an effect of, or a contributing cause of, several health conditions. Talk to your doctor if you are at all concerned about, or are experiencing symptoms of, any of the diseases discussed here.

CHAPTER 5:

ANDROPAUSE: FACT OR FICTION?

LET'S REVIEW. WE'VE DISCUSSED THE FUNCTION and importance of testosterone, some of the ways and reasons that it decreases, and what some of the noticeable symptoms of that decrease are. By now it should be clear that for healthy men, the drop in testosterone begins sometime in the mid 30s to early 40s, is quite gradual, and typically doesn't drop so low as to stop outright the ability of a man to father children or function sexually.

However, at around midlife, that gradual decline, accumulated over 15 years or so, cause some men to display some of the symptoms of testosterone deficiency, including loss of interest in sex, fatigue and depressed mood, irritability, and difficulty concentrating, that are rather similar to the changes that a woman of about the same age experiences when she goes through menopause. And thus, in recent years, a new term has forged its way into the media and health-related lexicon: "male menopause." And like any health topic that receives considerable media attention, male menopause has received considerable *marketing* attention as well, in the form of books, over-the-counter supplements, and prescription treatments.

But is it really the equivalent of the female menopause, or is it just more junk science, another instance of a buzzword condition propagated to sell patches, pills, and creams? If you're reading this book, odds are that you're concerned that you might be experiencing so-called male menopause, and that you might be considering treatment to relieve its symptoms. In this chapter, we'll try to separate the fact from the volumes of fiction out there surrounding this often controversial topic.

First, though the term male menopause has earned household-name status only within the last decade or so, scientists have been studying it for about 60 years, only way back when, they referred to it as "the male climacteric." Studies started appearing in medical journals in the mid 1940s.[23] The term andropause would be coined about a decade later.

Fast forward to 2005, and the term andropause may not exactly be fodder for cocktail-party conversation, but has, along with its more common name of male menopause, become more or less familiar to the general population. The truth behind it, however, has not. The important question here is (a) does testosterone drop in such a way as to mirror the precipitous drop in estrogen, and eventual cessation of reproductive capabilities, that women go through during menopause, and (b) does that drop in testosterone create enough of a health problem to warrant medical treatment? The answer to the first part of the question, for the average healthy male, is "no." The answer to the second part is "sometimes." Whereas menopause is inevitable for all women who live past their childbearing years, andropause for men is not. And while the jury is still out on issues surrounding hormone replacement therapy for post-menopausal women, the jury is yet to even enter deliberations on the clinical implications—if any—for declining testosterone in the aging male.

The other question is whether and when to call it andropause. The word andropause is derived from the root words "andro," which, you'll remember, comes from the Greek for man, and "pauein," from the Latin, meaning to cause to cease. So then, andropause can be called by its rightful name only when the body has ceased production of testosterone (and other androgens). This, as we discussed in the last chapter, usually happens only in cases of the surgical removal of the testicles, as in the case of those with testicular tumors, some men with prostate cancer, and male-to-female transsexuals, and in cases where there is severe injury to the structures of the brain that signal the testicles to produce testosterone. This may sound similar to hypogonadism, which you may recall is defined as reduced or absent secretion of testosterone. But while all hypogonadism is andropause, not all andropause—as it's commonly described—is hypogonadism. (And even then, a very small amount of testosterone is still produced by the adrenal glands.) What we can say with a fair degree of certainty is that yes, andropause does exist, but no, it is not a normal part of the aging process in the same way that menopause is in women.

So, will the *real* medical terminology please stand up?

You might remember from chapter 2 the quiz commonly administered by doctors called Androgen Deficiency in the Aging Male, or ADAM. Symptomatic ADAM, or Symptomatic Late-Onset Hypogonadism (SLOH) are the much more appropriate common terms used to describe the gradual decline in testosterone that comes with normal aging. Symptomatic is the key word here. Yes, all men will produce testosterone in increasingly shorter supply with each passing year, starting around the mid 30s to early 40s, but not all men will become symptomatic—at least not to the point where they may want to seek relief from those symptoms. And even among those who do experience symptoms, not all of them are necessarily candidates for testosterone replacement therapy.

However, popular culture being what it is, the term andropause has come to be used interchangeably with ADAM and SLOH, even though they dramatically differ. To keep things simple let's stick to one term. I'll use SLOH throughout this chapter to mean a drop in testosterone, as a result of normal aging in a healthy man, which is presenting some of the common unpleasant symptoms associated with that drop.

SLOH: How Do You Know?

The ADAM questionnaire is a great way to start the screening process for men who may have SLOH, but it is by no means the be all, end all. One of the problems is that the symptoms don't always come neatly packaged together at the same time, and at the same degree of intensity. Furthermore, because testosterone declines naturally over several years, the symptoms can come on so gradually that a man doesn't even know he has them—or he may notice them, but attribute them to other things, such as the effects of stress, workload, or just "getting older."

Another problem with questionnaire testing is that the symptoms described in it also happen to be the symptoms of several other things. Loss of energy, difficulty concentrating, and sexual difficulties are indeed symptoms of SLOH, but are at the same time some of the common symptoms of depression, for example. Or if a man already has been diagnosed with depression, and is taking antidepressant medicine, then some of its side effects, including sexual difficulties, may contribute to a misdiagnosis of SLOH.

Therefore, diagnosing low testosterone for a man over 40 requires something more thorough than the questionnaire. We discussed testosterone testing in chapter 2. In chapter 3, we learned that the fact that you have symptoms of low testosterone doesn't always mean that your body isn't producing a sufficient amount. Instead, much of it may be bound to certain proteins, and therefore not bioavailable or free—that is, it may not be able to reach the various androgen receptor sites where it's needed.

To recap, total levels of 300 ng/dL are the bottom end of the healthy-levels spectrum. Anything lower than 200 likely indicates some kind of a problem, whether it's an injury, a genetic factor, or SLOH. Your primary care physician should be able to measure your testosterone levels if you suspect SLOH may be the problem. But if you think your primary care physician may have misdiagnosed you, ask for a referral to a urologist, who will be more familiar with the symptoms of SLOH.

A Word on Erectile Dysfunction

Testosterone drops with age and so does, for about half of all men, the ability to achieve an erection. It is therefore commonly assumed that erectile dysfunction is caused by testosterone deficiency. This assumption is both incorrect and potentially hazardous to your health. The truth is that for the 50% of men over the age of 75 who have erectile dysfunction, some underlying disease or the effects of advanced aging is most likely to be the cause, and not low testosterone.[24] In fact, low testosterone is thought to be a very rare contributor to erectile dysfunction. While a strong enough libido is required for naturally achieving an erection (and that's testosterone's primary contribution to an erection), the physiology of an erection is more about basic hydraulics than sex drive. (This is why some men who take drugs to treat erectile dysfunction report feeling like they've solved only half the problem. Many men have the sex drive, but no erectile capability, and for them, Viagra, Levitra, or Cialis are a godsend. But many other men lack both sex drive and erectile capability, meaning that a drug-induced erection won't necessarily increase interest in sex.)

More often than not, the most likely culprits in erectile dysfunction are certain diseases whose likelihood also increases with age, including high blood pressure, diabetes, and artherosclerosis, to name a few.

The Low-Down

Comparing a man's steady decline in testosterone to menopause is pure semantics. There is simply no such thing as "male menopause." That said, there is a recognizable set of symptoms that accompany diminishing testosterone, which a man may or may not want to address. Call it what you will, but here's the low-down.

- Every man's testosterone declines with age, but not every man will experience it in the same way. Some men go well into their 80s with the strength and energy of a 20-year old.
- Symptomatic Late Onset Hypogonadism (SLOH) is a more accurate description of a *set of* symptoms relating to low testosterone.
- The symptoms associated with decreasing testosterone are also the symptoms of other health problems as well. If you are approaching your doctor with concerns, he or she will likely perform a complete work-up. If not, ask him or her to do so.

PART 2:

GET THE TESTOSTERONE EDGE

IF YOU'RE A REASONABLY HEALTHY MAN OVER THE age of 30, you may be inclined to conclude that you've effectively received a life sentence to watch helplessly as the very essence of your manhood wanes year after year.

Not so.

So far in this book we've focused on understanding the health issues surrounding testosterone: what it is and does, why it's important, and how production rises and falls throughout life.

In the next six chapters we'll be taking an inside look at current thinking on medical and lifestyle-based treatment of lowered testosterone—or at least the symptoms of lowered testosterone.

We'll examine five key areas where you may have the opportunity to stabilize or even reverse the effects of a natural age-related dip of testosterone levels: exercise, diet, dietary supplements, medical testosterone replacement, and overall lifestyle factors, including stress management.

There may not be a heck of a lot you can do (legally, anyway) to boost your testosterone levels, but there are plenty of things you can do boost your energy and mood, fight disease, and increase your sexual vitality. Getting *The Testosterone Edge* is more about adopting a better attitude toward your health and well-being than it is about increasing the amount of any single hormone in your bloodstream.

Your future health and happiness await. So let's begin.

CHAPTER 6:

TESTOSTERONE REPLACEMENT THERAPY

JOHN IS A 37-YEAR-OLD MAN WITH KLINEFELTER Syndrome (see chapter 3), a genetic condition where the man has an extra copy of his X chromosome, which—among other things—typically entails below-normal testosterone production. As a result, John has been on testosterone therapy (a gel that he rubs onto his arm daily) since he was 19. However, having been married for two years, and ready to consider parenthood, he spoke with an endocrinologist, who told him that a Klinefelter patient on testosterone therapy will not produce enough sperm for successful conception. In fact, he would need to go off testosterone for 6 to 12 months in order to see the desired results. (Testesterone replacement doesn't aid the body in producing the hormone. Instead, it takes over the process outright and sometimes creates an overabundance of testosterone. As we discussed in chapter 1, this can diminish LH production to the point where the body doesn't pick up the signals to produce sperm, thus making testosterone replacement an effective contraceptive.)

"I've been off testosterone for nine months now, and I've been tested three times for sperm analysis, and all three times, there was no sperm," he says. "Even when I was taking testosterone—no sperm."

Aside from that disappointment, John has, over the last nine months, become hypogonadal. "When I went off testosterone," he says, "I have to offset the effects by working out pretty aggressively. And I have to take calcium supplements—four big horse pills—every day. I've all but lost my sex drive, and I don't quite get erections. And the volume of ejaculate is very low—almost nonexistent.

"And I've gained a lot of fat. After nine months, it's like I don't even have muscles. My performance in weightlifting is the same. I can lift the same weight, but I look different."

John says that before this, the longest he had been off it before was for six weeks. "And when I went back on, I was 'horny as a billy goat.' I feel depressed when I don't take it. Things affect me more. I feel down, and sad. There's something a bit off in the emotional element."

He says that though he's excited by the possibility of becoming a father, he can't wait to go back on testosterone. "I'll be on it for life, until they tell me I can't take it. It makes me feel more alive, more confident," he says.

Whether you think you may currently be experiencing low testosterone, or are concerned that you may in the future, the question of medical testosterone replacement therapy (TRT) is bound to come up. It may even be the main reason you picked up this book to begin with. And if the numbers are any indication, you're far from alone. According to IMS Health, Inc., a company that tracks the pharmaceuticals industry, the number of patients using TRT grew by 29% in 2002.[25] And the Mayo Clinic reports that pharmacies filled 2.2 million testosterone prescriptions in 2003—twice the number filled in 2000.[26]

Problem is, the number of men lining up for TRT is growing faster than the body of scientific research examining its long-term safety, and when it should be prescribed. (The figures cited above provide no indication of the diagnoses for which those prescriptions were filled.) Let this chapter be your introduction to TRT, including the current medical debate, and also the various options for TRT delivery.

TRT Comes of Age

You might remember from chapter 1 that TRT, or something like it, goes way back. Whether it was the half-baked "therapy" of animal-testicle-extract injections in nineteenth century France, or some of the truly bizarre remedies of the ancient world—how'd you like your doctor to prescribe ingesting animal testes as a cure for impotence?—it seems that treating the natural waning of the male hormone has long been of interest. But it wasn't until around the 1930s when modern TRT as we know it came to be. That was when scientists were first able to isolate the hormone and produce a synthetic version of it—and not a moment too soon. Just prior to this discovery, animal and human testicle transplants were gaining momentum.

Synthetic testosterone replacement soon became a widespread treatment for truly hypogonadal men, and later it would come to be considered a medically valid treatment for the symptoms of SLOH. However, it would be about 60 years until public interest in the idea of TRT to relieve the symptoms of aging for average men would surge. There might be a couple of reasons why this is so. To begin with, as I've mentioned several times so far, men, unlike women, do not experience a precipitous drop in hormone levels during their fourties or fifties. All men will experience a decline in testosterone levels, but only in rare cases do they drop significantly enough to be of medical concern. Second, because the decrease is so gradual, at about one percent per year, most men don't notice a sudden change, and even when they seek medical attention for the symptoms, it's often misdiagnosed as depression, stress, or simply "aging." And third is the sociological element—the macho attitude (which, ironically, is often attributed to testosterone) that many men maintain, less than willing to admit that their bodies are no longer producing the same amount of the very stuff that makes them men.

But fast-forward to the 1990s, and men began to listen to the claims of drug companies touting the benefits of TRT as a sort of fountain of youth, a means of reversing the course of nature, of reclaiming lost muscle, vitality, and libido.

The Controversy

John, from the beginning of this chapter, is a case of a man whose body produces an unhealthily low amount of testosterone. His muscle mass decreases and his bones become brittle without his testosterone therapy. Testosterone therapy isn't a bed of roses. John needs to have his hormone levels checked frequently, along with his prostate. But without it, he'd be unhealthier than he would be otherwise.

Remember from chapter 5 that only under relatively rare circumstances does a man find himself in this situation. In cases of damage, infection, or disease to either or both testicles, or in cases of Klinefelter syndrome (like John's) and certain other diseases, the body cannot produce sufficient testosterone to maintain bone density, muscle mass, and sexual function. This is considered true hypogonadism. For these men, there is no question that testosterone replacement therapy works. If a man has almost no testosterone, and is administered testosterone therapy, then it will effectively stop or reverse many of the attendant symptoms.

For the average, reasonably healthy man over age 30, though, it's a different story altogether. In the typical older male, testosterone is likely to have declined, but not to a worrisome degree, only an undesirable one. Again, many men can and do remain sexually active, and even father children, well into their seventies and even eighties.

Before we take a more detailed look at some of the most popular medical and non-medical treatment options, it's important to have at least a cursory understanding of the current debate surrounding treatment for symptoms of SLOH. You might remember from chapter 2 that many doctors feel the normal decline in testosterone that healthy, aging men experience is a quality-of-life issue rather than a medical one. This is still a topic of lively debate in medical circles. Adding to the problem is, as we discussed earlier, the difficulty in diagnosing SLOH.

The heat in this much-heated debate comes from the question of whether otherwise healthy men over the age of 35 should consider testosterone replacement in the same way that otherwise healthy postmenopausal women may consider hormone replacement therapy. What's also subject to debate is whether testosterone replacement therapy can even treat many of the common symptoms of normal testosterone decline. (We'll leave out of this discussion the topic of healthy young men using testosterone supplements in order to enhance physique or athletic performance.)

Many in the medical community wonder if the recent popularity of TRT is just another example of the pharmaceutical companies "medicalizing" the otherwise normal effects of aging. In other words, are we moving toward a trend of treating the average older man for a disorder that exists only as a matter of semantics? And if so, what if any, long-term consequences are in store?

In 2002, the National Institute on Aging (NIA) and the National Cancer Institute teamed up to request that the Institute of Medicine conduct a 12-month study to review and assess the latest research regarding the possible risks and benefits of TRT for otherwise healthy older men.

The IOM committee concluded in its report that, with the exception of clinical trials to learn more about its safety, TRT should be limited to its only FDA-approved indication: true hypogonadism. (As we'll discuss in later chapters, this standard has also affected women. In 2004 the FDA refused to approve Procter & Gamble's testosterone patch for post-menopausal women.) Through the report, the IOM made five major recommendations,[27] which are paraphrased below.

1. Conduct clinical trials. A clear benefit should be established before assessing any long-term risk of TRT for older men with low testosterone.
2. Begin with short-term, randomized, double-blind placebo-controlled efficacy trials. The participants should be 65 and older and have testosterone levels below the physiologic levels of young adult men.
3. Conduct longer-term studies if short-term efficacy is established. Studies to determine long-term risks and benefits should be conducted only if clinically significant benefit is established in the initial trials.
4. Ensure the safety of participants.
5. Conduct further research, particularly regarding age-related changes in testosterone levels.

In response to the IOM report, the NIA issued the following statement:

> [A]lthough some older men who have tried these treatments report feeling "more energetic" or "younger," testosterone therapy remains a scientifically unproven method for preventing or relieving any physical or psychological changes that men with normal testosterone levels may experience as they get older. Except for a relatively few younger and older men with extreme deficiencies, testosterone treatment is not deemed appropriate therapy for most men at this time.[28]

So there you have it. Well actually, maybe not. After all, a lack of sound scientific backing, and caution from experts have never stopped Americans before from doing things that are potentially hazardous to their health. It seems we'll do just about anything to look or feel better, and non-medical TRT has apparently joined the ranks of tanning booths, plastic surgery, and diet pills.

Treatment Options: Pros and Cons

While the controversy over testosterone replacement therapy will likely continue for many years to come, one thing is for sure: the number of healthy older men taking testosterone—inconclusive research be damned—has nearly tripled in recent years, grossing some $400 million for the drug companies each year.[29] Perhaps it's the alluring prospect of effectively turning back the clock and reclaiming lost youth. Perhaps it's in response to genuinely decreased quality of life brought on by naturally declining testosterone. Either way, the long-term results just aren't known yet.

Actually, that's not entirely true: Researchers have determined that testosterone delivered in pill form impairs cholesterol metabolism. Because the pill is taken orally, it is metabolized by the liver, just like everything else you swallow, and may lead to both benign and malignant tumors.[30] And, based on some smaller short-term studies, researchers do have preliminary evidence on the possible pros and cons of testosterone replacement. The possible pros should be obvious: they are the improvements in muscle and bone mass, libido, and mood that sometimes accompany drooping testosterone.

In 2004, Ernani Luis Rhoden, M.D., and Abraham Morgentaler, M.D., published in the prestigious *New England Journal of Medicine* the results of their review of the most recent research, assessing the suggested risks of testosterone replacement therapy. Below is a review of some of those possible risks described in that article.[31]

Coronary artery disease. Because men have higher testosterone than women, and also have higher instances of heart disease than women, some have suggested a link between the two, and that testosterone replacement increases that risk. However, no research to date has shown any direct connection between heart disease and testosterone replacement. In fact, testosterone therapy may even have a beneficial effect on the risk of cardiovascular disease by improving lipid profiles. As a secondary effect, it may also provide the energy to engage in increased physical activity.

Prostate enlargement. During puberty, the presence of testosterone signals the prostate gland to enlarge. That growth levels off after puberty, but starts back up again at middle age. Problem is, this gland, primarily responsible for making semen, surrounds the urethra. The larger the prostate gets, the more of a chokehold it puts on the urethra, often to the point of impeding or completely blocking the flow of urine. About half of all men over 50 have a condition known as benign prostatic hyperplasia (BPH), a symptomatic but non-cancerous growth of the prostate, which makes urination more frequent and less forceful. Many men with BPH find themselves awakening during the night with the need to urinate.

Because testosterone signals prostate growth, testosterone replacement is likely to increase the volume of the prostate gland, especially during the first six months of treatment. However, little evidence exists to suggest that the prostate necessarily grows to the point of triggering BPH symptoms. At best, researchers conclude, some men may occasionally experience such symptoms.

Prostate cancer. Remember from chapter 2 our example of men with prostate cancer undergoing therapy to reduce testosterone? Some have suggested that if low testosterone helps fight prostate cancer, then supplemental testosterone must put men at higher risk. This has been difficult to prove. As risk of prostate cancer increases with age, it's hard to tell if the 70-year-old man diagnosed with prostate cancer (and who had been receiving testosterone replacement) would have developed the cancer regardless of testosterone.

Based on the latest research, it appears that the risk of prostate cancer for those undergoing testosterone replacement therapy is about the same as for the general population. In other words, there is no compelling evidence to date that it causes prostate cancer.

Testicular atrophy or infertility. This is a real and very common risk, especially among younger men receiving testosterone replacement treatments. Testicles usually become smaller and softer, and fertility rates are typically greatly diminished. These effects are usually reversible with cessation of treatment, and many men will likely need to cease treatment for months or even years before preparing to conceive.

Skin reactions. Not a serious health problem, but about 60% those who receive transdermal testosterone treatment in the form of a patch experience a rash at the site. Of those who use a rub-in gel, 5% experience such symptoms. Also, a small number of men experience oily skin and acne, similar to that of a pubescent boy.

Male-pattern baldness. No evidence exists to support a link, although increased body hair is sometimes reported.

Fluid retention. When the body retains fluids, blood volume increases, meaning that the heart has more blood to pump, making its job harder. It also increases the workload of the kidneys. Fluid retention resulting from testosterone replacement therapy is rare and very mild when it does occur. However, researchers suggest caution when prescribing testosterone to patients with congestive heart failure or renal insufficiency.

Sleep apnea. Sleep apnea is a condition in which the muscles surrounding the airway relax during sleep to the point of blocking the airway, causing the sufferer to wake gasping for air. Some people who have apnea may wake up as many as 100 times during the night! Further, these frequent awakenings usually prevent the sufferer from staying asleep long enough to achieve rapid eye movement and slow-wave sleep—the deep stages of sleep required for full rest and recovery from the day.

There appears to be a slight risk of developing sleep apnea for men who (a) are treated with higher doses of testosterone and (b) already present some of the other risk factors for the disease, including the following:

- Being male (the disorder is three times as prevalent in men)
- Smoking
- Being overweight or obese (indicated by a neck circumference of 17 or more inches)
- Heavy drinking

However, the dimensions of the upper airway appear unaffected by testosterone replacement, which suggests that any breathing problems have their roots in "central mechanisms" (the working of the brain and nervous system that regulate respiration) rather than anatomical changes.

Polycythemia. In chapter 2 we discussed the mild anemia that many older men experience as a result of lower testosterone. Starting at puberty, testosterone raises hemoglobin levels, and those levels taper off in tandem with the gradual decline in testosterone as we age. Polycythemia is anemia in reverse: an overabundance of red blood cells. The condition can have unpleasant side effects—headaches, dizziness, skin irritation—or dangerous consequences, including a higher risk of high blood pressure and blood clots.

Men receiving testosterone replacement will see a mild rise in red blood cells, which is generally beneficial. However, researchers have determined a risk of higher-than-desirable levels for some men. They have determined the risk to be greatest among men who receive injections, with 43.8% of patients having a documented elevation of red blood cells. However, these instances were considered mild and of short duration, with no serious consequences. Furthermore, testosterone delivered through a gel or a patch showed a much smaller risk. Research does suggest caution for men who have a pre-existing condition that could be worsened by the presence of higher red blood cell count, such as chronic obstructive pulmonary disease. But to date, no testosterone-related instances of blood clots have been reported.

Breast swelling. A small number of men undergoing testosterone replacement therapy report breast tenderness and swelling; stopping treatment will usually reverse it. It's likely that this affects mostly men who are overweight or who are abusing synthetic androgens. As you'll recall from chapter 3, high concentrations of body fat often lead to aromatase activity, in which testosterone is converted to estrogen. Similarly, synthetic androgens are often converted to estrogen.

Know Your Medical History

Because testosterone can affect pre-existing medical conditions, or interact negatively with certain medicines, or alter body chemistry in such a way as to pose the potential for health complications, it's vital to have a full medical history taken before your doctor prescribes testosterone replacement therapy. Before using testosterone in any form, tell your doctor if you have a history of the following. (And if you don't know, and are concerned that you might, ask to be tested.)

- ***Liver problems*** (especially important if you are a candidate for an oral-delivery form of testosterone, which is metabolized by the liver).
- ***Prostate problems***. The cells of the prostate are responsive to testosterone, and may enlarge in the presence of increased testosterone, causing difficult, frequent, weak, and nighttime urination. Also, while testosterone replacement hasn't been shown to *cause* prostate cancer, men with pre-existing prostate cancer should absolutely not receive testosterone replacement.
- ***Heart problems***. There is some debate in medical circles whether testosterone protects or hurts the heart and circulatory system.

Until a final verdict is delivered, it's better to play it safe, and tell your doctor about any preexisting condition or family history.

- ***Diabetes.*** Testosterone may, or may not, change insulin dependence for the better. Even so, any unexpected changes in blood glucose levels can be unpleasant or even harmful. If you have type 1 or type 2 diabetes, make sure you discuss those concerns with your doctor.
- ***High cholesterol level.*** In somewhat rare cases, testosterone replacement in men can unfavorably tip the balance of HDL and LDL cholesterol. If cholesterol levels have been a problem in the past, be sure to say so.
- ***Sleep apnea.*** Because testosterone is known to contribute to sleep apnea, those who currently suffer from the condition ought to be on high alert.
- ***Allergies to medication.*** Obvious enough, and your doctor will likely ask you about your history of medical allergies, but do make sure to mention any past known reactions to any medicine.

An Introduction to TRT Methods

What follows is a brief introduction—a primer, if you will—on the various methods of delivery for testosterone therapy. Time was when intramuscular injections were the only delivery method considered safe. The problem with injections is (a) well, they're injections, and (b) they result in a sharp rise in testosterone shortly after administration, followed by a steady decline to baseline, pre-injection levels, until it is time for another dose. Patients receiving injections are on a hormonal rollercoaster ride of ups and downs. Nowadays, injections are still around—and the technique has improved—but other delivery methods have been developed.

Oral Buccal Delivery

Typical dosage: 5 mg, 10mg, or 25 mg tablet (usually taken at least twice a day)

Covered by insurance? Every insurance company is different, but generally, yes, for approved uses

Out-of-pocket expense: Depending on dosage and insurance coverage, $5 to $30 per month

Buccal (pronounced "buckle") is an oral delivery method of medicine designed to dissolve in the mouth. It is typically taken by placing the dose between the cheek and gums of the upper mouth by your canines. (It should never be chewed or swallowed.) The most commonly prescribed brand-name buccal testosterone delivery is Striant.

Buccal testosterone is made to be taken twice a day, usually at 12-hour intervals. In addition to the side effects of androgen replacement generally, buccal testosterone carries the risk of these unique side effects:

- Irritation, redness, pain, or swelling at the application site
- Infection of the gums
- Change in how food tastes or an unusual taste in the mouth

Pills and Capsules

Typical dosage: 0.625 mg to 2.5 mg, once daily
Covered by insurance? Yes, for approved uses
Out-of-pocket expense: $30 to $40 per month

By and large, pills and capsules are falling out of favor because of evidence of potential harm to the liver. Damage is usually associated with prolonged administration of high doses. However, brand-name caplets like Testred remain on the market.

Topical Gel

Typical dosage: 2.5 mg to 6 mg per day
Covered by insurance? Yes, for approved uses
Out-of-pocket costs: $5.00 per month

Topical testosterone gel is applied to the skin, and delivered steadily into the bloodstream, typically over a 24-hour period. It is usually applied either to the shoulders, upper arms, or abdomen, and is sometimes applied to more than one site with each dose. The brand names most popularly prescribed for this delivery method are AndroGel and Testim.

Because topical gel contains alcohol, it dries quickly on the skin. That also means that it is highly flammable, so smoking or cooking with gas shortly after application is strictly prohibited. Also, because it is applied to the skin, there is the potential for transfer to another person who touches that skin area. This is especially important to consider if you make frequent physical contact with a woman who is or may be pregnant. Exposure to gel can cause complications with the pregnancy Because it is rubbed into the skin by hand, it is also important to thoroughly wash your hands with soap and water after application to prevent transfer to others. There's no known optimal time frame to wait before swimming or showering after applying a topical testosterone gel, but one manufacturer advises that it is reasonable to wait five to six hours.

Transdermal Patches

Typical dosage: Up to 30 mg, designed to enter the bloodstream at a rate of 2.5 mg to 6 mg per day
Covered by insurance? Yes, for approved uses
Out-of-pocket costs: $5 per month

Similar to a topical gel a transdermal patch is applied directly to the skin, either on the back, arm, buttocks, leg, abdomen, or scrotum. (Some makers recommend changing the application site each day for some men.) The most commonly prescribed brands of transdermal patches are Testoderm and Androderm.

In addition to the general risks of androgen replacement, patches carry the risk of these unique side effects or complications:

- Rash or irritation at the site of application
- Patch falling off when the skin sweats

Intramuscular Injections

Typical dosage: 25 mg to 200 mg, depending on its form and the patient's needs
Covered by insurance? Yes
Out-of-pocket costs: $5 per month

Injections may be administered by the doctor or the patient, provided he has proper training. As mentioned earlier, injections result in an immediate surge of testosterone, followed by a steady decline leading up to the next injection, which normally takes place 30 days from the last injection. Aside from being somewhat painful and inconvenient (if the patient needs to go to a doctor to receive injections), the dosing is highly inconsistent, considering the 30-day roller coaster of sharp highs and deep lows. Injectable testosterone is still available and widely prescribed to those who, for one reason or another, are not candidates for other delivery methods, such as those who have severe skin reactions to topically applied testosterone. The post popularly prescribed brands of injectable testosterone are Delatestryl, Everone, Tesamone, Testro, and Virilon.

Jeff's Story

Jeff Altman is a 54-year-old man from New York. When he and his second wife had begun trying to conceive, there had been difficulties. After repeated attempts he admits that, almost as an afterthought, he considered that "Maybe it wasn't her problem; maybe it was mine." A lab test showed that he was producing almost no testosterone at all. "My doctor actually asked me if I'd had a vasectomy," he says. (It should be noted that a vasectomy does not affect testosterone.) "I thought there was a lab error. It was shock." Even today, Jeff and his doctor haven't been able to determine why his testosterone is so abnormally low, but he suspects that it's been an issue for nearly the last 20 years of his life.

In the meantime, they had adopted a child. As Jeff tells it, "Energy was a big issue. I had a young son who always wanted to play, and I had no energy. I was perpetually fried—and my concentration was gone too, which had implications for home and work."

After much consideration and many discussions with his wife, Jeff decided to consider TRT. His wife was concerned about the potential side effects, including the possibility of transmitting some testosterone to her through body contact.

Jeff tried the patch (placed on his buttock), but found it to burn, and has instead been taking testosterone for two years in gel form, applying it to his shoulder and abdomen. The first time he took it, as he tells is, "Within ten minutes, the lights started coming back on in shocking fashion. My concentration is so much better. My sex drive is clearly back, and the 'ogle factor' has improved."

One of the side effects for Jeff is that, due to an enlargement of the prostate, he has noticed an increased frequency in urination; he often wakes up during the night to empty his bladder. However, he works closely with his doctor to monitor his symptoms every six months.

Side effects notwithstanding, says Jeff, "I feel like I'm the poster child for [TRT]. So many guys walk around not knowing where their energy and drive went. We're told that it's just 'getting older,' but there may be legit medical conditions that aren't normal. A man who's not feeling as he did before should go to his doctor if he's not comfortable with it."

Other Possible Side Effects

While researchers are still hard at work to determine the possible long-term effects of testosterone, some more or less short-term side effects are already recognized, and in fact are indicated by the drug manufacturers themselves.

Drug interactions

Depending on the dose and the person receiving it, testosterone replacement may interfere with the following medicines:

- **Anticoagulants:** Some forms and derivatives of testosterone have been reported to decrease the anticoagulant requirements of patients receiving oral anticoagulants. Those who are on oral anticoagulant therapy require close monitoring, especially when androgens are started or stopped.
- **Oxyphenbutazone:** This is an anti-inflammatory drug used to treat arthritis and bursitis. Taking it along with testosterone may increase the blood levels of oxyphenbutazone to potentially undesirable amounts.
- **Insulin:** Insulin-dependent diabetics (those with type 1 diabetes) may notice a decreased requirement for insulin. That's not necessarily bad news, but it is important for any diabetic to be aware of the possible effects of any new medical treatments on blood glucose.

Fluid and electrolyte disturbances

Testosterone replacement has been shown to promote retention of sodium chloride, water, potassium, calcium and inorganic phosphates. Fluid retention can lead to increased blood pressure. Potassium imbalance can cause muscle cramps or spasms.

Generalized side effects

Just about any prescription medicine, especially when a patient begins using it, can produce the generalized side effects of introducing a foreign substance to the body. Testosterone is no different, and documented generalized side effects include the following:

- Nausea
- Headache
- Nervousness or anxiety
- Diarrhea
- Dizziness
- Dry mouth
- Insomnia
- Decreased libido
- Bronchitis
- Abnormal ejaculation

Other Uses for TRT

When a drug is prescribed for purposes other than those originally intended, that's called "off-label" use. It's a fairly common practice with some drugs, and testosterone is one of them. Here are some of the off-label uses currently in use for testosterone.

Depression. As we've discussed several times already, the effects of lowered testosterone often mirror the effects of clinical depression, and many men are often diagnosed as having depression, and are treated with antidepressant medicine. However, in the days before antidepressants, testosterone therapy was a conventional treatment for men seeking relief from depression. It hasn't been until recently that some doctors have considered whether testosterone deserves a second look as a depression treatment.

A recent small study conducted at McLean Hospital, in Belmont, Massachusetts tested the effectiveness of testosterone gel on 56 men with depression who had not responded as they had hoped to conventional antidepressant therapy. Some of the men were given a placebo and some were given a relatively low dosage of testosterone gel; all continued their antidepressant regimen. At the end of the eight-week study, those on testosterone had reported significant improvements based on several standardized measurement scales for depression. (One of the men noticed increased difficulty urinating, which reflects the increased prostate size that is often a side effect of the treatment.)[32]

Inducing puberty in adolescent-aged boys. Late onset puberty is a condition in which boys of puberty age do not experience the physical changes

Is There a Backdoor to Testosterone Replacement Therapy?

IN THE NEXT CHAPTER we'll take a look at all kinds of supplements that claim to boost testosterone, but don't involve a direct infusion of real or synthetic testosterone into the body. Rather, they are "precursors," meaning that they enter the body with a particular chemical makeup, but the body then converts them to testosterone. (Whether that actually happens is another story, and something I discuss in the next chapter.) Aside from anabolic steroids, the supplements in the next chapter are available to just about anyone with enough money and proximity to a health-food store—or Web browser.

However, there is one alternative treatment that's gaining interest among bodybuilders, but is available only with a doctor's prescription. Clomiphene citrate (sold under the brand names "Clomid" and "Serophene") is a drug used for fertility treatment in women. It works by inducing ovulation and acts as an anti-estrogen, which tricks the brain into producing more fertility-friendly follicle-stimulating hormone and luteinizing hormone.

That anti-estrogen property is what makes it interesting to some men. Men too produce a small amount of that "female" hormone, but blocking its production could—*could*—mean a proportionately higher level of testosterone. However, medically speaking, there isn't a lot of interest in this form of treatment. There's no reason to think a backdoor approach would be any safer or more effective.

of puberty. It can happen for one of three reasons: a "constitutional delay" (a family history of "late bloomers"); an underlying medical problem, including diabetes, cystic fibrosis, kidney disease, asthma, or even malnutrition; or problems with, or damage to, the testes, pituitary, or hypothalamus.

Testosterone treatment for this condition typically consists of a four-month program of testosterone injection treatments but may be ongoing in the case of Klinefelter syndrome or other congenital condition.

AIDS-Related Wasting Syndrome. Diminished muscle mass accompanies the ravages of AIDS. Further, the disease itself often contributes to a lowering of testosterone. The majority of studies have found testosterone replacement (whether prescribed in conjunction with a muscle-building exercise program) halts, or at least significantly slows, this wasting of muscle mass.

The Low-Down

More than likely, the debate over testosterone therapy will rage on and on over the next couple of decades. There's a lot we don't know yet, but here's what we can say for sure:

- Testosterone therapy has several known side effects, and it should not be taken by those with certain physical conditions such as sleep apnea and prostate cancer, among others
- Testosterone replacement is available only with a doctor's prescription, and each delivery method has its own pros and cons—and risks, in some cases.
- The most current thinking is that testosterone should be prescribed in medically necessary cases, not simply as a "quality of life" drug.
- At present, not enough research has been done to truly assess the long-term risks and benefits of testosterone replacement.

CHAPTER 7:

SUPPLEMENTS AND OTHER ALTERNATIVE TREATMENTS

IN 2005, STEROIDS WERE A HOT-BUTTON ISSUE, attracting plenty of attention from the government and the media. Baseball star Jose Canseco had published his book, *Juiced: Wild Times, Rampant 'Roids, Smash Hits, and How Baseball Got Big,* which painted a none-too-flattering picture of the world of professional athletes using performance-enhancing substances (some of them illegal) to set world records and inspire legions of young athletes to do "whatever it takes" to be just like them. In the following weeks, Congress held hearings on performance enhancers, on the heels of a ban in October of 2004 on some "prohormone" supplements.

But attention to performance-enhancing supplements is nothing new. Some historians think that athletes from as far back as ancient Greece (and maybe even earlier than that) used any manner of concoctions—though nothing like what's available nowadays—to give them the competitive edge in sports and in life.

In this chapter we'll take a look at some of the herbal, nutritional, and hormonal supplements (some of them illegal) out there that claim to boost testosterone, or at least provide some of the desired effects of increased free testosterone levels, including increased muscle mass, a revved-up libido, improved mood and physical energy, and improved ability to sustain concentration.

Sounds pretty good, doesn't it? It does for a lot of men who aren't candidates for medical replacement, but want to stack the deck in their favor toward higher testosterone production and usability.

But let's take all of this with a big note of caution. So far, much of the evidence out there, as you'll see, isn't terribly convincing. Some supplements have shown promise, but mainly because they have the ability to correct a nutritional imbalance that had previously kept the body from functioning as it should. Others may show some benefits because they have stimulating properties, but nothing that a good old-fashioned cup of coffee couldn't handle.

The majority of studies show no significant increase in testosterone levels, and many show some downright scary side effects, especially when it comes to anabolic steroids and yohimbine (a preparation derived from tree bark, which we'll discuss below).

The supplement industry is, of course, an industry, bent on making money. Many popular supplements have been blamed for misleading marketing, and describing their benefits in technically correct, but obscure, language. For example, walk into your average vitamin shop and take a look at some of the so-called muscle-building powders on the shelf. Many of them claim to have "anti-catabolic nutrients, muscle-cell volumizers, and insulin potentiators." Sounds pretty scientific, doesn't it? Well, do you know what those three things are? They're none other than your old familiar friends, vitamins, water, and sugar! Other supplements claim benefits based on their containing substances that actually are contained in the pill (or powder, or drops, or whatever), but are converted into something else altogether by the time your body is done processing them. It's kind of like those brands of instant oatmeal claiming to be a good source of vitamin C. Stuff in the package *does* contain vitamin C, and so the makers are allowed to claim as much, but the vitamin is destroyed the second you pour boiling water on it. Similar idea here.

And here's one more little bit of supplement-ese I'd like to translate for you. From time to time you'll see that supplements include "orchic extract." Care to guess what that means? It's the extract from animal testicles! You might remember from chapter 1 our friend Charles Édouard Brown-Séquard injecting himself and others with "liquide testiculaire" as a remedy for aging. Archaic though it may seem, the practice is apparently still *en vogue* today after all—and still just as bogus.

When it comes to bold claims and big promises attached to high price tags, be sure to do your homework before you take a supplement. Almost no herbal supplement is regulated by the Food and Drug Administration. (In fact, the Administration went so far as to state that, as far as over-the-counter herbal aphrodisiacs are concerned, none work to treat sexual dysfunction.) That means that, not only are there no standards for safety, but between manufacturers, the methods of extracting and preparing the supplements, along with the recommended dosage to achieve the desired effect, vary widely. So even when a particular herb *does* have some scientific backing behind it, that doesn't mean that the herbal preparation you're taking will necessarily provide the same results.

And lastly, many supplements you may be tempted to take may very well interfere with any prescription medicines you currently take. You've heard it a million times before, but you're going to hear it here again: talk to your doctor before you go experimenting on yourself.

Let's take a look at the substances in this chapter based on their claims to fame. Understanding that many are backed by claims of multiple benefits—increased libido *and* erectile capabilities, for example—we'll categorize each by the primary benefit associated with it. The categories we'll look at are:

1. Increased testosterone (a literal increase in total or free testosterone in the blood)
2. Increased libido
3. Improved or regained erectile ability
4. Improved mood or mental clarity

For clarity and simplicity, any substances that also claim to increase strength and muscle mass as a primary benefit (performance enhancers) are discussed in the first category.

Substances Claiming to Increase Testosterone

The following substances claim to directly increase total or free testosterone, or indirectly increase testosterone by converting to testosterone as part of a metabolic process or by improving your body's ability to produce testosterone.

Anabolic Steroids

You know that testosterone is a steroid hormone. So technically speaking, you have steroids in your bloodstream at the moment. However, the term steroid has become almost universally associated with the injectable, performance-enhancing kind, known as anabolic steroids. Officially speaking, they ought to be called anabolic-androgenic steroids, but for simplicity's sake, let's go with the familiar term.

An anabolic steroid means any drug or hormonal substance, chemically and pharmacologically related to testosterone, other than estrogens, progestins, corticosteroids, and dehydroepiandrosterone (DHEA, see below). Steroids are illegal unless prescribed by a doctor, and they can have negative, and even fatal, effects if abused. Those side effects include liver tumors and cancer, jaundice, high blood pressure, kidney tumors, severe acne, trembling, atrophy (shrinking) of the testicles, reduced sperm count, infertility, and female-style breast development. (And those who abuse the injectable form also run the risk of contracting communicable diseases, including HIV from sharing needles.) Sounds like a real hoot! So why take them?

Athletes and bodybuilders are drawn to anabolic steroids because there's little doubt that they significantly increase muscle size and strength, much more so than any human could ever achieve through diet and exercise alone. The steroid gives the body a ridiculous surge of testosterone-like effects which, combined with diet and exercise, produces almost superhuman results. (It doesn't, however, increase testosterone levels per se. As with testosterone replacement, those who take steroids don't supplement, but replace, their body's natural production.)

However, the people who take anabolic steroids are *not* superhuman, and so they're susceptible to the many serious side effects of steroid use, including stunted growth (if taken during adolescence), acceleration of tumor growth, enlarged prostate, acne and oily skin, female-style breast growth, and changes in blood pressure, to name but a few.

Bottom line: don't even think about it.

Human Growth Hormone

Human Growth Hormone (HGH) is a chemical messenger secreted by the pituitary, and is vital for growth during childhood and puberty, and also for daily repair of normal body wear and tear. Just as with testosterone, your body produces less and less HGH as you age, starting in the early 30s.

HGH therapy has been available for some time, whether through an injection or through supplements taken orally. It is designed to help those whose growth has been stunted—usually due to some disease of, or damage to, the pituitary gland—but a trend toward "off label" use for the therapy (to slow down the aging process and to increase muscle and bone) has researchers concerned. Furthermore, while the "improvements" in muscle and bone among those who inject HGH are undeniable, several studies failed to assess muscle strength, only size. That means that these changes may have been functionally irrelevant. Further still, even with scant research, several side effects are known (and likely several more will be discovered) associated with the therapy, including arthritis-like pain, joint swelling, changes in blood sugar, and liver damage, among others.

Several over-the-counter supplements that claim to perform the same work as HGH are available. While these products do not contain HGH (which is available only by prescription), they are a combination of amino acids and, because each manufacturer his its own "secret recipe," there has been no research to validate claims made by any single combination found in any such supplement.

Androstenedione

This supplement received a fair deal of popular press about five years ago, but it's all moot at this point because the Food and Drug Administration successfully banned androstenedione (a.k.a. "andro") in October of 2004, labeling it a "controlled substance." Nowadays, anybody possessing andro without a prescription faces fines and up to two years in prison.

Androstenedione is a "prohormone," a chemical precursor to testosterone. Because pure testosterone is illegal without a doctor's prescription, supplement makers were quick to market andro and other similar supplements as kinder, gentler—and legal—alternative to steroids. For years andro flew under the radar, popular mainly among the bodybuilding set, until in 1998 it was discovered that baseball superstar Mark McGwire was taking the supplement during his record-breaking season. Sales exploded among bodybuilders, athletes, and ordinary civilians. (Many critics of the ban blame McGwire for drawing attention to andro, and thus dragging the substance into a wider government debate on performance-enhancing supplements.)

Even with McGwire's record to back its claims, the fact remains that andro doesn't have the same effects as testosterone, and like DHEA, is often converted to estrogen. Furthermore, one of its side effects appears to be lower levels of HDL ("good") cholesterol.

DHEA

Dehydroepiandrosterone, or DHEA, is a steroid hormone, in the same way that testosterone and estrogen are. Like testosterone, it begins its life as cholesterol. The body makes its own DHEA in the adrenal glands, and lifetime production peaks at around the mid-twenties, before a steady decline, following a path similar to that of testosterone. (DHEA will increase testosterone in a truly hypogonadal man, but isn't guaranteed to do anything in normal men.)

To this day, researchers are still not entirely clear as to exactly what DHEA does in the body, but some researchers have noticed a connection between abnormal levels of DHEA and obesity and insulin resistance. Also, most agree that because of its similarity to testosterone and other hormones, it is easily converted to other hormones. That fact alone has fueled the marketing hype behind DHEA supplements (derived from plants) as an anti-aging miracle pill, providing the same basic effects as testosterone. By taking DHEA supplements, you're not taking testosterone, but—or so the argument goes—you're setting your body up to convert the DHEA into testosterone. And apparently, it's working—the marketing, that is. DHEA is widely touted in athletic circles (among body builders especially) as a performance enhancer, a magic pill that can turn back the clock, boost sex drive and mental function, burn fat, build muscle, and provide a competitive edge.

But where's the beef?

The Food and Drug Administration has remained up in the air over the last decade as to how to even classify DHEA. In the early 1990s DHEA supplements were sold as weight-loss pills, but the Agency forced makers to stop selling it. Then in 1994, it was reclassified as a dietary supplement (technically a food, not a drug), which allowed for it to be sold over the counter.

While it is available over the counter, it has been banned among several athletic organizations, including the International Olympic Committee, National Football League, and National Basketball Association. (Baseball is the only professional sport that still allows it.)

Although vitamin shops and Web sites sell bottle after bottle of the stuff to athletes and fountain-of-youth seekers alike, no credible study has proven that the supplement does what it say it does: significantly increase testosterone. In fact, one study[33] conducted in 1999 suggests

The Untouchable DHEA?

If DHEA is a steroid hormone, and is banned by several sporting agencies, then why is it, like androstenedione and other supplements, not banned from sale to the general public? That question was at the center of a major debate in the early spring of 2005, when the *New York Times* published an editorial stating that Republican Utah Senator Orrin Hatch, had lobbied hard to keep it off the list of banned substances. Why? Because, the newspaper claimed, Utah is where many makers of vitamins and supplements, including DHEA, are based, and the senator sought to protect his state's industrial and economic interests.[34] (With several other supplements having been banned, sales of DHEA rose sharply.) And what's more, the senator's own son is a lobbyist for the National Nutritional Foods Association, a trade association for the dietary supplement industry.

Hatch fired back in a letter to the editor, saying that Congress had given the Drug Enforcement Administration the authority to schedule DHEA as a controlled substance, and that "the same law that exempted DHEA based on its past history of beneficial use—and lack of evidence of abuse—also changed the criteria for adding to the controlled-substances list."[35]

that it has virtually no effect on testosterone. The researchers examined the effects of eight weeks of DHEA supplements on young men. The men, all in their twenties, were divided into two groups. The first group was given 50 mg of DHEA daily. The second group took 150 mg daily and followed an eight-week weight training program. The researchers concluded that "Serum concentrations of free and total testosterone...were unaffected by supplementation and training....These results suggest that DHEA ingestion does not enhance serum testosterone concentrations."

So while DHEA can be converted into other hormones, which *can* in turn be converted into testosterone, that doesn't mean that they necessarily *are*. As a matter of fact, it is often broken down into estrogens. Furthermore, DHEA supplements are not without their side effects. Again, the research is inconclusive, but some of the commonly reported side effects include baldness, acne, prostate enlargement (in turn leading to frequent, weak, and nighttime urination), and irritability and restlessness. And because DHEA is often converted into estrogen, one possible side effect is female-style breast growth and other feminizing characteristics.

Tribulus Terrestris

Also known as "puncturevine," tribulus terrestris is an herb from Bulgaria that has caught on among bodybuilders in recent years. It's believed to stimulate the production of luteinizing hormone, which in turn signals the production of testosterone. It has also been used in several cultures for other purposes for centuries, including as a mood enhancer, and for the "fortifying" of the liver and kidneys.

In a study conducted in 2000[36] researchers broke a group of men up into those who would take a daily dose of tribulus terrestris equal to 3.21 mg per kg of body weight, and those who would take a placebo. Body composition, body weight, diet, and overall mood were evaluated in all subjects before the trial, in which all participants entered an eight-week resistance training program. At the end of the program, the researchers found no changes in body composition, body weight, and mood among either group, leading them to conclude that tribulus terrestris does not enhance body composition or exercise performance.

ZMA

A combination of zinc, magnesium, and vitamin B6 (among other ingredients), ZMA may be one supplement to show some level of promise, but we're still being cautious. A study published in 2000[37] divided a team of 27 college football players into two groups: one that took a ZMA pill every evening before bed, and one that took a placebo. Both groups participated in their college athletics during the trial. The study was said to be "double blind," meaning that neither the players nor the people collecting the data knew what the purpose of the study was (which helps ensure unbiased reporting of the data.)

At the end of the study, those who took the supplement saw an increase in total testosterone from 567.92±131.96 ng/dL to

752.17±141.08 ng/dL. Free testosterone (the testosterone not bound in the blood) rose from 132.10±36.16 pg/dL to 176.34±36.11 pg/dL. (Those who didn't take the supplement saw a drop in free and total testosterone probably due to excessive exercise.)

Though the study was double blind, and published in a peer-reviewed journal, you should be aware that one of the study's authors, Victor Conte, is the inventor of the ZMA supplement. That fact isn't necessarily damning, but judge for yourself before you wholeheartedly agree with research published by someone who has a significant financial stake in a positive outcome.

Chrysin

Chrysin is a compound known as a flavonoid, and is believed to be a natural aromatase inhibitor, meaning that it blocks the enzymes that tell testosterone to convert to estrogen. That's not the same thing as increasing the body's testosterone production, but the idea of keeping what you have is nothing to sneeze at, especially as you age. Chrysin occurs naturally in various plants, including the *Pelargonium* species, which are germanium-like plants; the *Passiflora* or passion flower species, which include tropical passion fruit; and the *Pinaceae* species, including pine trees. (These sources are used to produce chrysin in its concentrated-extract form.) It is also abundant in honey and propolis, a substance that bees produce to make their hives.

Early studies suggest that supplemental chrysin is not absorbed well into the bloodstream, so while the stuff in the caplets may indeed have aromatase-inhibiting powers, it'll never be put to use. (Some manufacturers of chrysin supplements claim to have "solved" this problem by adding additional extracts, believed to help the body absorb and utilize chrysin.)

One recent study from Italy[38] measured urinary testosterone levels of male participants in a 21-day program of eating foods known to be high in chysin at levels consistent with a supplemental dosage. There were no changes in testosterone levels after 7, 14, and 21 days of treatment, as compared to baseline values or to study participants who did not change their diet. The researchers concluded that "the use of these foods for 21 days at the doses usually taken as oral supplementation does not have effects on the equilibrium of testosterone in human males."

Nettle Root Extract

Extract from the nettle root (a.k.a., Urtica dioica L, a.k.a., "stinging nettle") have been used for decades in Europe to combat the effects of benign prostatic hyperplasia, an enlargement of the prostate gland, which is non-cancerous, but nevertheless often unpleasant, as it contributes to frequent, weak, and nighttime urination.

In recent years, some have suggested that nettle root extract can (in a way similar to chrysin) help your body to make full use of the testosterone floating in your bloodstream. You'll remember that there's a difference between your total testosterone and the free testosterone that's available to affect the androgen receptor sites of the body. What keeps some testosterone from being free is sex-hormone binding globulin (SHBG), which attaches to testosterone. Nettle root extract is believed to have an "affinity" for SHBG. That means that when it's introduced into the blood stream, it, rather than testosterone, will attach to SHBG, which in turn frees up more testosterone.

Not much research has been done on the effects of nettle root extract on SHBG or free testosterone. One often-cited study[39] is widely touted as "proof" that nettle root supplements work. Researchers isolated or semi-synthetically produced the various compounds in the plant collectively known as lignans, which are thought to bind to SHBG. In test-tube studies, the researchers found that all lignans, except for one, developed a "binding affinity" to SHBG in the test tube. (One lignan, divanillyltetrahydrofuran, was found to be "outstandingly high" in its binding affinity.) But because the study was conducted in test tubes there's no evidence that it would produce the same results if ingested. No further credible studies have looked at the effect of ingested nettle root for these purposes.

On the other hand, its effects on increasing urinary flow and decreasing urinary frequency are fairly well documented. That in turn could reduce nighttime awakenings, thereby increasing sleep time and energy, and decreasing anxiety about the symptoms of benign prostatic hyperplasia, both of which could in turn have a positive effect on libido, mood, and strength.

Sarsaparilla

You probably know sarsaparilla best as the stuff that makes root beer taste the way it does. In fact sarsaparilla is the very root that root beer refers to. But it's also been used to treat a wide variety of conditions—even though it hasn't been proven effective in treating a single one. It's been used as a "cure" for syphilis, and as a treatment for epilepsy and tuberculosis, among others.

More recently, it has been hyped as testosterone booster, probably because the root actually does contain compounds with a steroid-like chemical structure. However, these compounds do not produce steroid-like effects in the human body, and no studies have validated claims that sarsaparilla has any effect at all on libido, muscle mass, or erectile function.

Substances Claiming to Boost Libido

The following are substances with claims to increase the level and frequency of interest in sex or sexual activities.

AVENA SATIVA

If you've ever heard of "sowing your oats" as a metaphor for libido-fueled behavior, then you're familiar with the centuries-old affiliation between oats and virility. (Notice that nobody says he's going to sow his wild apples!) In recent decades, some concentrated oat extracts, including avena sativa, have been marketed as an aphrodisiac in general and a testosterone booster specifically.

Avena sativa is more commonly known as green oats. Though it's been used medicinally for hundreds of years, no published studies have documented any of its purported benefits. However, promoters say that avena sativa frees up bound testosterone in the blood, making it more available to be taken in through the body's androgen receptors, rather than remaining bound in the blood. Most of the benefit associated with it is cited from research conducted in the 1980s by the Institute for Advanced Study of Human Sexuality, which—wouldn't you know it—also happened to market its own line of avena sativa products. However, the research was never published in a credible medical journal, and besides, the results of the very small study (only six people were involved) were too erratic to be taken seriously.

SAW PALMETTO

The berries of the saw palmetto tree have been used for years (mostly in Europe, but it's been catching on the U.S.) to improve urine flow by weakened non-cancerous enlargement of the prostate called benign prostatic hyperplasia, a condition that affects almost half of all men over 50. Saw palmetto does this by inhibiting the conversion of testosterone to something known as dihydrotestosterone (or DHT for short), a metabolic product of testosterone that contributes to the rapid cell growth—and thus overall enlargement—of the prostate. However, this is a relatively limited effect. (It may also aid in keeping DHT from binding, and in excreting DHT from the body.)

Though its folk-use history, beginning in the Native American tribes, originally touted it as being good for virility, there's no credible evidence that it has any directly positive effect on libido. That said, many men with benign prostatic hyperplasia often wake up throughout the night to urinate, leading to chronic cycles of fatigue. Improved sleep likely leads to improved mood and increased energy, both of which can have an indirect effect on libido.

Pygeum

Pygeum is an herb that originates from southern Africa. It contains plant sterols, which have a steroid-like chemical structure, but in this case produce no steroid-like effects, such as increased muscle mass or improved libido.

Like saw palmetto, pygeum is used nowadays mainly to lessen the symptoms of non-cancerous prostate enlargement. Researchers believe that it can help due to a natural anti-inflammatory effect, and also by ridding the prostate of cholesterol deposits that can accompany a benign prostatic enlargement.

Damiana

Damiana (Turnera Aphrodisiaca) is widely used—as its Latin name would suggest—as an aphrodisiac. The yellow-flowering shrub was first used by the Aztec Indians, and has been used in the U.S. since the late 1800s.

While it enjoys a rich and storied folk history for its libido-boosting properties, any effect it may have likely comes from the fact that it acts as a mild stimulant, which can improve mood and increase interest in sex. (It's also sometimes used for depression, and to address the emotional and hormonal symptoms of PMS.) However, no scientific study to date exists to show that damiana mimics any testosterone-like effects in humans.

Eurycoma Longifolia Jack

Eurycoma Longifolia Jack (a.k.a. tongikat ali) is native to Malaysia and has a long history among Malaysians as a libido booster and sexual enhancer. It is believed to have stimulant effects and also to promote production of luteinizing hormone, which in turn plays a role in testosterone production.

No human studies exist to support these claims one way or another. What few studies do exist were performed on rats and—curiously—the majority of these studies were performed by the same researcher. One such study[40] examined the sexual qualities of middle-aged male rats after they received a daily dose of Eurycoma longifolia Jack during a 12-week period. The results showed that the dose enhanced the sexual qualities of the middle-aged male rats by decreasing their hesitation time, which, said the researcher, "further supports the folk-use of Eurycoma longifolia Jack as an aphrodisiac."

Ginseng

Ginseng is almost legendary in its reputation for treating and preventing several diseases. It's one of the oldest medicinal roots known. Its history stretches back millennia to ancient China.

Among its purported qualities is that of a sexual enhancer for both men and women. The root does display a mildly stimulating effect, not unlike caffeine, which increases physical energy and enhances mood. However, no hard evidence exists as to a positive direct effect on human sexuality.

Substances Claiming to Improve Erectile Function

Erectile dysfunction is often the result of several factors working simultaneously. As I've mentioned before, testosterone may play only a bit part in the body's ability to achieve an erection strong enough to sustain intercourse. However, erectile dysfunction (diminished or lost ability to achieve and maintain an erection) often coincides with age and decreased testosterone. The following substances claim to improve erectile functioning.

L-arginine

Widely touted in its supplement form as a "natural Viagra," L-arginine is an amino acid that occurs naturally in several foods, and is necessary for the body's formation of nitric oxide, which is essential for achieving an erection. However, there is no such recognized medical condition as an L-arginine deficiency.

Most studies have looked at L-arginine as part of a combination treatment for mild erectile dysfunction, so its specific role or effectiveness is not clear. A study of 30 men with erectile dysfunction tested a commercially available treatment preparation sold under the name ArginMax. Twenty-five subjects diagnosed with mild to moderate erectile dysfunction were evaluated over a 4-week period while on ArginMax, but only 21 completed the study. Of them, 19 showed an improved ability to maintain erection during sexual intercourse.[41]

A larger study[42] looked at 45 men with erectile dysfunction, who took a combination of L-arginine and herbal preparations one to two hours before intended sexual activity. The results were promising—so much so that the researchers concluded that "on-demand oral administration of the L-arginine…combination is effective in improving erectile function in patients with mild to moderate [erectile dysfunction]. It appears to be a promising addition to first-line therapy for [erectile dysfunction]."

Yohimbine

Yohimbine has a long folk history as a libido enhancer, and more recently as a testosterone booster and performance-enhancing treatment. This substance, derived from the bark of a tree native to Africa, has been the subject of no scientific research to support claims that it increases testosterone or produces testosterone-like effects.

It may, however, be somewhat effective in treating erectile dysfunction. "Somewhat" is the key word. Most major clinical studies have tested yohimbine as part of a combination of two or more treatments, so it's difficult to parse out how effective—or ineffective—it is. One thing's clear though: It's never been shown, on its own or as part of a combination therapy, to be nearly as effective as mainstream medical treatments. If you're drawn toward more natural treatments, you may be interested to know that yohimbine shows more potential negative side effects than its mainstream counterparts. Part of the way it may work to improve libido and erectile function is in its mildly stimulating effect. (The stimulating effect is part of the reason it's often included in over-the-counter "metabolism-increasing" weight-loss formulas.) However, even taken at standard dosage (a maximum of 40 mg in a 24-hour period), this stimulating effect can lead to dizziness, nausea, insomnia, anxiety and panic, rapid heartbeat, and a spike in blood pressure. Exceeding standard dosage can have serious effects, including loss of muscle function, vertigo, and even hallucinations. Judge for yourself, but I'd recommend extreme caution with yohimbine.

Muira Puama

Muira puama (a.k.a., "potency wood") comes from the stems and roots of the ptychopetalum olacoides plant. It's been used for generations as an aphrodisiac and is also believed to have other medicinal uses, including treatment of erectile dysfunction.

Virtually no research evidence exists to support claims that muira puama does as it claims. The few published studies have been small, or did not pass muster in terms of scientific validity. Anecdotal evidence would suggest that men who take it have reported improvements in their sex drives and erectile strength and frequency. However, it is unclear whether this is the result of a placebo effect.

Substances Claiming to Improve Mental Functioning and Mood

Testosterone is believed to play a role in cognitive functioning and the ability to maintain concentration. Cognitive functioning and concentration can be impaired by several factors in addition to low testosterone, including diet, fatigue, emotional factors, medication, injury, and others. Below are two substances that claim to improve these mental qualities.

Ginkgo Biloba

The ginkgo tree originated in China and later spread to Korea and Japan. Nowadays, you can find it just about anywhere, a testament to its hardiness and adaptability, which may help to explain why it is the oldest of all surviving tree species. (Darwin is said to have called the tree a "living fossil.") Ginkgo biloba, an extract prepared from the pointy leaves of the ginkgo tree, has been used for years to treat a variety of conditions, including dementia. Its supplemental form has been popular in recent decades—especially in Europe and the United States—improving mood and cognitive function and preventing so-called "senior moments." Of course, depressed mood, lack of mental focus, and inability to concentrate are also symptoms of low testosterone, so any validation of claims to boost mental function is of interest to us. On the other hand, much of the research to date on ginkgo (and there isn't much) is conducted on animals or on those with severe depression or cognitive impairment, as is the case with Alzheimer's disease.

One study looked at the use of ginkgo in reasonably healthy subjects as a general quality-of-life enhancer and cognitive function improver. Sixty-six volunteers between 50 and 65 submitted to a 4-week program of taking either 240-mg doses of ginkgo biloba or a placebo. Before, during, and after the trial, the subjects were asked to complete multiple questionnaires to assess their overall quality of life, and also completed tests to gauge motor performance and mental functioning.

Though the actual percentages of increase are not clear, the researchers found that the group that took the ginkgo biloba rated themselves higher in their subjective assessments of their mental health and overall quality of life, and that they scored higher on the motor and cognitive tests.[43]

One of the other common folk uses for ginkgo biloba is in treating erectile dysfunction. Among ginkgo's effects is that of decreasing the "stickiness" of blood platelets, and thereby having a thinning effect on the blood. (And for that reason, it should not be taken along with aspirin, another blood thinner.) The improved blood flow is believed to lend to improved erectile functioning in men who take the supplement. This is especially so for men whose lifestyles have resulted in impaired blood flow, such as those who smoke, have diabetes or heart disease, or have high cholesterol—all of which have been linked to erectile dysfunction.

However, to date no convincing studies exist to suggest a direct physical erectile response to ginkgo biloba supplements in reasonably health men. Some tests have been conducted on those who have developed sexual dysfunction as a result of taking a certain class of antidepressants, and even those studies show mixed results (although most of them do suggest a slight improvement as a result of the treatment.) Erectile dysfunction, of course, is often more complex than the mere hydraulics of erection, and is often caused by some balance of physical, mental, and emotional difficulties. Ginkgo has been more effective as a mood enhancer and cognitive-function improver, both of which could very well have an indirect effect on erectile function.

CAFFEINE

Caffeine is the most widely used drug on the planet, and here in the United States, more than 80% of us consume it every day. While the main method of delivery is of course a good ol' cuppa joe, other major sources are soft drinks and tea. It's also found in some headache medicines and in chocolate, both of which are also consumed daily by many Americans.

While most people who consume caffeine regularly do it to "jump-start" themselves in the morning and to boost flagging alertness in the mid-afternoon, it has also proven itself beneficial in improving cognitive functioning. (Because of the "buzz" of energy it provides, it's also been used as a performance enhancer, but no studies confirm any impressive gains in muscle strength.) In one study,[44] subjects were divided between those who habitually used caffeine and those who did not. Within each group, subjects consumed either caffeine or a placebo. Before, and then 30 minutes after consumption, subjects were asked to complete computerized testing, subtraction tasks, and a sentence verification task, and to gauge their moods based on a subjective scale. The researchers found that for both groups, following the caffeine, there were significant improvements in simple reaction time, numeric working memory reaction time, and sentence verification accuracy. Both groups also showed a reduction in self-rated mental fatigue, and significant improvements in alertness.

It may sound great, and for the most part it is—which probably partly explains why the vast majority of us are regular caffeine consumers. Just be careful to use it in moderation. One or two cups of coffee, or the equivalent, a day ought to be your limit. (And by cup, I mean eight ounces, not those gigantic tanks of the stuff that have become so popular.) Too much will disrupt sleep, which will have the opposite effect on mental functioning, and may also lead to dependency on caffeine.

Other Alternative Approaches

Many Americans, for one reason or another, will try an alternative approach to a health problem before accepting a conventional medical treatment. In fact, in 2002, nearly 75% of Americans reported having tried some form of complementary or alternative medicine at some time, and 62% reported having done so within the prior 12 months.[45] Exactly what qualifies as an alternative remedy is a matter of debate. Some may say that many of the supplements we've just covered are alternative remedies, and there's some truth to that claim. Others may argue that, because herbal medicine predates conventional western medicine by millennia, modern medicine is the true alternative. Still others argue that certain treatments, like hatha yoga, may have healing qualities, but are not alternative medicine—just a good idea.

Semantics aside, for the purposes of this section, we'll focus on some alternative approaches to low testosterone that do not involve orally administered preparations: specifically, hatha yoga, transcendental meditation, bright-light therapy, and acupuncture.

Hatha Yoga

Throughout the late 1990s yoga enjoyed a wild resurgence in popularity, with yoga studios popping up across the country faster than you can say "downward facing dog." The history of yoga stretches back (no pun intended) millennia—as far back as 7,000 years by some records—to ancient India. The word yoga is Sanskrit for "union," and practitioners believe that a lifetime of following yogic teachings is a path to unifying mind, body, and spirit.

The term yoga actually refers to several paths to such union. Some involve prayer and meditation. Some involve service and devotion. The one you're probably most familiar with is so-called "hatha" yoga, which combines physical poses with deep breathing and mental concentration. "Power yoga," "ashtanga yoga," and other styles are simply varying approaches to hatha yoga.

The benefits of hatha yoga, when done safely and properly, are well recognized in even the mainstream medical community. They include stress management; improved flexibility, strength, and muscle tone; improved sleep and digestion; and increased concentration. Several poses, most of them variations of a cross-legged sitting posture, are said by some to increase the production and release of testosterone. Clearly the ancient yogis didn't know what testosterone was, so one must assume that this is an updated explanation of an ancient claim to boost masculinity and virility. But when it comes to claims like that, don't believe the hype. There's no evidence at all that sitting, bending, folding, or twisting your body into various shapes has any effect at all on your body's testosterone production.

That said, the stress-relieving element of regular yoga practice can counter the ill effects of excessive stress on testosterone production.

Transcendental Meditation

Transcendental Meditation is a copyrighted meditation technique taught by Maharishi Mahesh Yogi, and is practiced by over five million people worldwide. This simple form of meditation involves the repetition of a word (a mantra), and each practitioner is given a unique mantra by his or her instructor.

Many people are attracted to Transcendental Meditation ("TM," for short) because it requires no particular belief system and is fairly easy to learn. And like yoga, its stress-relieving and alertness-enhancing effects may counteract the effects of stress on testosterone.

No widely accepted studies have been performed to show a direct effect on testosterone production, but researchers at the Center for Health and Ageing Studies at the Maharishi University of Management in Indiana do claim to have performed studies showing a direct improvement. Researchers at the university studied four hormone levels in test subjects—cortisol, growth hormone, thyroid-stimulating hormone and testosterone—before and after 4 months of either the TM technique or other forms of stress management. They found "significantly different changes for the two groups, or trends toward significance, for each hormone over the 4 months." The subjects who practiced TM showed decreases in basal cortisol level and rises in testosterone. (Exact levels of rise or fall aren't clear.) The researchers concluded that, "Overall, the cortisol and testosterone results appear to support previous data suggesting that repeated practice of the TM technique reverses effects of chronic stress significant for health."[46]

Bright Light Therapy

You might remember from chapter 1 that your body's testosterone production follows a predictable daily rhythm of highs and lows. Most biological functions do—everything including appetite, digestion, sleep, and body temperature. These so-called circadian rhythms were developed and hard-wired into the human body throughout the millennia as a way to better adapt to, and survive in, our environment. One of the environmental cues that is so important for regulating circadian rhythms is exposure to light. Our ancestors spent most of their time outdoors, and adapted to an environment where the position and intensity of the sun's light would change throughout the day. The rising sun meant the start of a new day, and the setting sun meant it was time to retreat to safety in order to go to sleep. (If you need proof of this effect, just try to sleep with the lights on!)

Fast forward to 2005. You have the same set of biological equipment that your ancestors had, but you don't have the same environment. We spend most of our time indoors, where we can make it light or dark at our choosing. Perhaps over the generations we will adapt to this as well, but biological adaptation happens much more slowly than human innovation.

A study by researchers at the University of California, San Diego School of Medicine[47] found that luteinizing hormone production was increased after exposure to bright light in the early morning. You'll remember from chapter 1 that luteinizing hormone is produced by the pituitary gland, and is essential for testosterone production. It was a small study of 11 men, but 5 days of bright light exposure (1,000 lux) in the early morning increased luteinizing hormone levels by nearly 70%, as compared to no material change when exposed to less than 10 lux.

Acupuncture

Acupuncture is, for all practical purposes, the longest-running clinical trial in the history of mankind. Its history reaches back to ancient China, and is based on a belief that "chi," the basic essence of all life, flows through the body through pathways called meridians. Blockages along those pathways, it's believed, are the root of illness, and stimulating those pathways through acupuncture clears up the blockages to restore health.

Nowadays, western science has taken a look and has noticed that the flow of bioelectricity through the body's nerve channels is very similar to what the ancient Chinese were describing some 5,000 years ago. Whether chi and bioelectricity are indeed one and the same is a topic of some debate.

Acupuncture hasn't been cited as a treatment for low testosterone, but it has been commonly used to treat depression and low physical energy, which correspond to low testosterone, with varying degrees of success.

An interesting study from the Netherlands was performed to test how acupuncture may treat erectile dysfunction.[48] Sixteen patients received acupuncture twice a week for 4 weeks. After treatment, the researchers measured urinary levels of testosterone, luteinizing hormone, and follicle-stimulating hormone. The results of the study were less than encouraging. Fifteen percent of the patients reported an improvement of the quality of erection, and 31% reported an increase in their sexual activity. No changes were noticed in hormone levels.

The Low-Down

There you have it. Supplements in a nutshell—or gel-cap, as it were—along with other alternative treatments for the symptoms of low testosterone. It goes without saying that the banned substances have no place in your regimen. Some of the others may, but aren't necessarily superior to conventional medical care. When it comes to using supplements to boost testosterone, or manage some of the symptoms of lower testosterone, here's the low-down:

- Talk to your doctor first. Just because some supplements are available over the counter doesn't give you a free pass to play doctor on yourself.
- "Natural" or "herbal" is not synonymous with "safe." Many naturally occurring substances can be dangerous at some dosages, and can also negatively interact with medicines you may take.
- Take it all with a grain of salt. Many of the benefits associated with some supplements are more folklore than hard science.
- Beware the placebo effect. Many bodybuilders and athletes swear by certain substances to help them build muscle—but they also spend countless hours in the gym, eat specialized diets, and may be genetically predisposed to higher performance and development. It's often quite difficult in these cases to parse out what—if any—effect a certain supplement is having.
- Alternatives such as yoga and meditation may help you to improve concentration, improve mood, and reduce irritability. (Yoga will also help improve strength.) Acupuncture may also help with mood, but likely doesn't have a significant effect on erectile function. Bright light therapy has shown some initially promising effects, but more research is likely needed to know for sure.

CHAPTER 8:

EXERCISE

ONE OF TESTOSTERONE'S IMPORTANT FUNCTIONS is to facilitate a certain level of muscle mass. So some people reason that the more muscular a person is, the more testosterone he must have. But that's not necessarily true, and in this chapter we'll explore the connection between muscle mass and testosterone, including how exercise can even *decrease* your testosterone levels. We'll also explore why exercising to increase your muscle mass can help to stabilize or even reverse some of the symptoms of the natural age-related decrease in testosterone.

Benefits of a Regular Exercise Program

First, though, here's my sales pitch for adopting an exercise plan in general. Don't skim over this section. You'll find that many of the benefits and precautions we discuss here will be directly applicable to how exercise and testosterone are connected.

Study after study indicates that exercise is as important for good and long-lasting health as a balanced diet, adequate sleep, and staying away from nicotine and excessive amounts of alcohol. In fact, it's been said that if exercise came in a pill it would be the most widely prescribed pill in the world. And yet, the Centers for Disease Control and Prevention report that well over half of all Americans are not active at a level that promotes health—even with new looser standards. The CDC now say that even things you wouldn't normally consider physical activity—sweeping the floor, making photocopies, "aimless wandering"—count toward the recommended minimum of 30 minutes per day.

It's reasonably easy to see why Americans don't exercise as much as they ought to. On the one hand, life has gotten pretty easy. There's a gadget or gizmo that can do in half the time, and with almost no effort, the tasks that would have kept your grandparents busy for the better part of the day. Dishwashers, clothing washers and driers, remote controls—yes, there was a time when these things didn't exist and people had to (*gasp*!) fend for themselves. Even the way we spend our free time requires less effort. In choosing between the La-Z-Boy and high definition TV (with a six pack of beer thrown in for good measure); and a stroll through the park or a game of touch football, it's all too obvious that most Americans choose the former.

On the other hand, life has in many ways gotten a little tougher. Americans are working longer hours than ever before. We're strapped for time. The average working adult may wake up at around 6:00 A.M., after five hours of fitful sleep, send the kids off to school, get ready for work, commute 45 minutes, work 9 or 10 hours, commute another 45 minutes back home, and pick up the dry cleaning and dinner on the way. At home, it's feed the kids, maybe catch up on some more work, do the dishes and laundry, and maybe catch 30 minutes of TV before tumbling groggily into bed, only to repeat the cycle again the next day. And we're supposed to find the time, energy, and motivation to exercise somewhere in the middle of all that?

Well, actually...yes. If you know what's good for you. If you have time to sit on your duff, watching *The Simpsons,* then you have time to get stronger and healthier. So let's take a look at all of those health benefits of getting off the sofa and into the action.

First, a word about exercise itself. Whether you're walking, cycling, lifting weights, or participating in a yoga class, all forms of exercise fall into one of two basic camps: aerobic or anaerobic. Aerobic exercise literally means exercise "with oxygen," meaning that increased oxygen intake is required to sustain the activity—as is the case with jogging, swimming, or cycling—because the oxygen is being used to help burn fuel. Anaerobic exercise, on the other hand, means "without oxygen." That doesn't mean that your body doesn't require oxygen during these kinds of exercises—just that it uses glucose as the primary fuel. Anaerobic exercises, like weight lifting or sprinting, bring the muscles to a state of high intensity and high rates of work for relatively short bursts. Because oxygen is not used, anaerobic exercise cannot last for long, and additionally, they create a byproduct called lactic acid, which contributes to muscle fatigue.

A good exercise program includes aerobic and anaerobic exercise, and flexibility training as well, all of which we'll cover later in this chapter. The benefits of exercise should be obvious enough to anybody who's ever seen a Bowflex infomercial. But those benefits extend well beyond the eye-popping pecs and lats. Let's take a look.

Strengthens muscles and bones. This seems obvious enough. In fact, most men are likely to begin exercise to strengthen muscles—or at least to increase muscle mass or improve muscle tone. Both types of exercise—aerobic and anaerobic—are important here. Aerobic exercise increases muscle endurance, while anaerobic exercise increases strength, while at the same time putting a moderate amount of stress on the bones, which causes them to strengthen.

Can maintain or change body composition. Remember, as you age, your body produces less testosterone, which will have an effect on your body composition, the ratio of fat to non-fat, or "lean mass." Sure, the numbers on the scale might not change, but your waist size might. Other factors come into play. As you age you'll also notice a decrease in metabolism, the rate at which your body burns calories while it's at rest. Furthermore, you might find that your overall lifestyle becomes less active in later years. You may omit some of the activity that had been built into your daily routine. You don't have to take this lying down. By consciously choosing to exercise on a regular basis, you can burn fat, build muscle (at any age!), and increase metabolism. Just look at Jack La Lanne, the man widely credited as the "godfather of fitness." Now in his 90s, the man has more strength and stamina than many men one-quarter his age—one-fifth, even!

Lowers blood pressure. Believe it or not, high blood pressure (a.k.a. "hypertension") is in almost every typical American's future. That may sound harsh, but it's true. Today, one-third of Americans have it, and new guidelines have classified previously safe numbers into a category called "pre-hypertension." We Americans, with our notorious diets and sedentary lifestyles are on a virtual collision course with this condition, which operates with such assassin-like stealth (it has no symptoms) that it has earned the moniker "the silent killer." Even a modest exercise routine can have a dramatic effect on blood pressure numbers.

Improves cholesterol and blood sugar levels. Exercise, especially aerobic exercise, increases HDL ("good") cholesterol, while lowering LDL ("bad") cholesterol, and also lowers triglycerides, which are linked to heart disease. And regular exercise has a definite protective effect against type 2 diabetes.

Decreases stress. Not that many of us need much motivation to want to decrease stress—it's just that so many of us go about it all wrong. Stress hurts. It chews you up and spits you out. It preoccupies your thoughts, disturbs your sleep, interferes with your daily activities, and has long-term effects on your overall health and well-being. But how do most people "deal with" stress? By doing many of the self-destructive things that lead to more stress down the road: overeating, abusing alcohol and other drugs, and relying on prescription or over-the-counter pills.

Exercise, on the other hand, is nature's stress buster, and anyone who's enjoyed a good workout at the end of a hard day will tell you that there's nothing quite like the calm, pleasant exhaustion after a good sweat. Taking it further, you may be surprised to know that stress has a demonstrated catabolic effect. That means that it eats muscle mass. The stress hormone cortisol is known to signal the body to use muscle tissue for energy and also to store extra fat. So in a very real way you can help to maintain your current level of muscle mass by decreasing stress. (In fact, I'd recommend exercise as only one part of a total stress management program that also includes relaxation techniques.) And furthermore, a well executed exercise program suppresses overall levels of cortisol.

Improves mood and mental function. Your mind isn't a muscle, but exercising your muscles can affect your mind and emotions in a profound way. As I mentioned above, exercise relieves stress. It can also dissipate anxiety, improve your body image, and boost your confidence in your body's efficiency and ability. Some studies also suggest that regular exercise can improve cognitive function. Either way, they don't call it a "runner's high" for nothing. Exercise is shown to help the body release the chemical messengers in the brain that support a sense of well-being.

Improves sleep. Sleep, glorious sleep! We all want more of it, and don't get enough of it. But sleep—and we're talking about deep, restful, restorative sleep here—is absolutely vital for feeling rested and maintaining good health. A number of diseases are linked to inadequate sleep, mainly because fitful, light sleep prevents the body from doing what it's meant to do during sleep: restore and repair itself. Sleep is the period during which the body releases growth hormones to repair and rebuild muscle. In one study published in the *Journal of the American Medical Association,* a group of healthy but sedentary adults 50 to 75 who had reported "moderate sleep complaints" were put on a 16-week exercise program. The exercise consisted mainly of 30 to 40 minutes of moderate-intensity walking four times per week. At the end of the study, all of the participants noted improvement in the time it took to fall asleep, the duration of sleep, and the overall quality of sleep, as measured by a self-rated questionnaire.[49]

The Muscle-Testosterone Connection

Let's get back to this idea that bigger muscles equal more testosterone. Certainly those pumped-up guys at the gym—you know the ones—who grunt and groan and flex in the mirror are much more "testosterized" than the scrawny teenager bagging groceries at the supermarket.

Au contraire.

Muscle mass is related to testosterone, but then again, it's related to a lot of other things, most notably, for our purposes, diet and exercise. More testosterone usually does equal more muscle (which is why boys pack on muscle during adolescence, the lifetime peak of testosterone production), but more muscle doesn't necessarily mean more testosterone—unless, of course, you're using anabolic steroids. In other words, testosterone is required for building muscle mass, but it's not sufficient on its own. Testosterone is produced through a feedback relationship between the testes, the adrenal glands, and the hypothalamus in the brain. The muscles don't play too prominent a role for the most part.

However, there does exist a connection of sorts, or at least physical activity has been shown to affect testosterone levels one way or another, even if only temporarily.

Both resistance training exercise (we'll call it weight lifting from here on), which is anaerobic, and aerobic exercise have been shown to increase testosterone, but only *during* exercise, and then only for about an hour or two afterward. After that it returns to normal resting levels, and even drops below resting levels if the exercise was particularly intense.

In a study published in *Medicine & Science in Sports & Exercise,* 10 healthy, but "untrained" (meaning non-athletic) men were tested before, during, and after they exercised on a stationary bicycle for 45 minutes, at 50% of their maximal oxygen uptake, a moderately intense level. After 15 minutes of exercise, both total and all-important free testosterone were "significantly increased...as compared to resting values."[50] And as expected, total and free testosterone dropped back to baseline within a relatively short period of recovery.

Another study compared how weight lifting affected the strength and total and free testosterone levels in middle-aged and older men. Two groups of men, the first with an average age of 46, and the second with an average age of 64, went on a 16-week program designed to increase the maximal strength and power performance of the arm and leg muscles. What's very interesting to note here is that both groups of men, even with the 20-year age difference, achieved significant gains in maximal strength and power output of the muscles trained. (Just goes to show that it's never too late to start exercising!) But no long-term significant increases in total or free testosterone were observed in either group. It even decreased a little among the 64-year-olds.[51]

Most studies have shown that neither weight lifting nor aerobics in and of themselves increase your testosterone levels over the long term. And as for why testosterone increases during exercise, researchers are still investigating that.

Too Much of a Good Thing

Plenty of research has shown that endurance-trained men, like marathon runners and long-distance cyclists, have lower total testosterone than sedentary men of the same age. Why this is true is still a matter of debate, but one European study took a look at the differences between a group of endurance athletes and sedentary men. Both groups were injected with gonadotropin-releasing hormone (which you might remember from chapter 1) to induce testicular testosterone production through the increased levels of luteinizing hormone. In both groups, testosterone production increased, but it did more so—almost twice is much—among the sedentary group.[52] Whether the suppressed production in endurance athletes is a permanent thing, or can be reversed by ceasing endurance exercise, is still undetermined.

How Exercise Helps

By now you're probably saying "Well, what's the point? If exercise alone can't increase my overall testosterone—and can actually end up *decreasing* it—then why exercise as part of my testosterone-enhancing plan?" This is where we get back to all those benefits of exercise. (See? I told you that you wouldn't want to skim over that section at the beginning of this chapter.) Exercise may not directly increase testosterone, but it can help you make the most of the testosterone you've got—which is nothing to sneeze at, considering that your testosterone levels are on the steady decline after age 30. The last thing you want is poor health (due to poor diet and exercise habits) making things worse.

Decreases Fat

Let's understand something: All weight loss is not created equal. When a person loses weight on a diet, much of that weight is fat and water, but up to 30% of the lost weight is muscle. Not good. Lost muscle in turn decreases metabolism (the rate at which your body burns calories while at rest), which sets you on a downward spiral: You won't be able to use calories as efficiently for energy, meaning that you'll have to diet more stringently in order to continue losing weight—or even just to keep from gaining weight. Could that be one of the reasons that most people gain back all of their lost weight (and then some) when they stop dieting? And adding exercise doesn't necessarily help. We'll discuss this a bit more later on, but some kinds of exercise may be good for your heart and lungs, but don't do much for maintaining muscle mass.

So "weight loss" is a misnomer in terms of what's desirable. It's not bodyweight itself that's important (heck, you could technically lose weight by having a limb amputated), it's the body composition idea we discussed earlier on: the ratio of fat tissue to lean mass. Perhaps "fat loss" is a better term. And as you'll remember from chapter 3, overweight and obesity is known to decrease testosterone. So losing fat (especially the fat that collects so stubbornly around your midsection) will help keep your testosterone from dipping. The older you get, the more important this will be, as older adults tend to put on fat more easily, due to an age-related decrease in metabolism. But building muscle increases your metabolism, which in turn helps prevents calories from becoming stored as fat.

May Decrease the Likelihood of Depression

Don't underestimate this. Depression is a very real testosterone sapper, and several studies have shown a positive link between exercise and preventing depression, or reducing and even reversing its symptoms in those who already have it.

And you might think that depression affects only a very small group of people, but you'd be wrong. According to the National Institute of Mental Health, every year approximately 18.8 million American adults (about 9.5 percent of the U.S. population age 18 and older) have a depressive disorder. Major Depressive Disorder (MDD), even though it's rarer, is in fact the number-one cause of disability in the United States and established and market economies worldwide. And on top of all that, depressive disorders often co-occur with anxiety disorders and substance abuse.[53]

A study conducted by Duke University Medical Center was performed on 156 people 50 and older who had MDD to assess the effectiveness of an aerobic exercise program compared with antidepressants. The participants were broken into three groups for a 16-week program: one group that would take antidepressants only, one group that would perform exercise only, and one group that would do both. At the end of 16 weeks, all groups had seen a significant reduction in depression, as measured by standard tests. Not only that, but there were the obvious secondary benefits, including increased aerobic capacity, and self esteem. The researchers concluded that "an exercise training program may be considered an alternative to antidepressants for treatment of depression in older persons."[54] I'm certainly not suggesting that if you're currently taking antidepressants you go off them. But this study demonstrates just how powerfully exercise can affect mood and well-being.

Do I Need to Join a Gym?

If you've never followed an exercise program before—or it's been a while since you have—you may think that getting started involves a membership to a health club, a personal trainer, and a closet full of spandex and expensive cross-training sneakers. Relax. You certain *can* go that route if you like, of course, but you could just as easily get a cheap set of exercise equipment from your local Sears—or even second hand. Or you could start with no equipment at all. That said, belonging to a health club can be a great motivator, and can add a social element to working out. Especially if you're new to (or returning to) exercise, maybe working with a trainer isn't such a bad idea, at least for the first couple of weeks.

In the end, it all comes down to what kinds of exercise you're going to do, and how much time and money you can put into it. (It doesn't make sense to join a gym if all you want to do is walk—you can do that for free!)

So let's take a closer look at what kinds of exercise can be of most benefit, and then have a look at putting together a program that works for you.

Getting Into the Act

The basic idea is this: balance weight-lifting exercises with aerobics in a way that helps you build muscle, lose fat, increase strength and bone density, and improve your heart and lung function. Most likely you can achieve that goal with three to five relatively short workouts per week. Remember, we're not talking about becoming gym rats here. Nobody ever said you'll have to spend hour after hour curling, squatting, jogging, or cycling. Your body doesn't ask for much.

You've no doubt heard this a million times before, but you're going to hear it here again: If you're new to exercise, or you're returning to it after a hiatus, or if you've been recently diagnosed with heart disease or any other medical condition, please talk to your doctor before beginning any exercise program.

The bottom line is that exercise is important for all men over 30, and not just because of testosterone. Get up, and get moving!

Strength Training Program

More muscle equals improved strength, increased metabolism, decreased fat, and more physical energy. Now here's the good news: most of what you think about strength training is probably *dead wrong*! Long, complex, ever-changing workouts may be what's needed to keep the material fresh in health-and-fitness magazines, but it's often quite unnecessary to help you improve your strength and build new muscle.

For this section on exercise, I've recruited the help of Pavel Tsatsouline, a former trainer to the Russian Special Forces, who now consults on strength training to the Navy Seals, the CIA, and elite athletes.

Pavel's theories and approach to exercise contradict much of what's found on today's "functional training" bandwagon. Forget about standing one-legged on a stability ball while doing a triceps extension. And forget about multiple sets of 12 repetitions. What follows may very well be the opposite of what you've come to think of as a strength- and muscle-building program. But if it didn't work, the Spetznaz, CIA, and Navy Seals, would have stopped using it long ago. When it comes to strength training, these are the dozen guidelines to live by:

1. Workouts should be short: 20 minutes or so.
2. Workouts should consist of a small number of "big" movements, involving multiple sets of joints, like deadlifts and presses, not a large collection of "little" movements like arm curls and leg extensions.
3. Workouts should leave you feeling refreshed and energized, not "spent" and sore.
4. Never—*ever*—work out to the point of muscle failure.
5. Workouts should consist of no more than three sets (including a warm-up set, if you feel the need to do one) of no more than five repetitions.
6. Cycle training is the absolute best way to increase strength (see below).
7. You can, and should, lift weights on consecutive days.
8. Weight lifts are to be executed slowly, deliberately, and with impeccable form.
9. Rest periods between lifting sets should be about two to three minutes.
10. Aerobics are important, but never aerobically warm up before weight lifting and always perform your aerobic training *after* your weight lifting sessions (it could be directly after, or later in the day, or on off days).
11. Strength is a skill, and workouts should be treated as practice sessions for that skill.
12. Strength is only as valuable as it is useful in a full range of motion. Flexibility is vital for getting the most out of your strength-training efforts.

But look around your average gym and check out the hardcore lifters spending hour after hour on multiple sets of high repetitions, and then bragging about how sore they are from their workouts. "Who cares how sore you are? The question is, 'are you getting stronger?'" Pavel said to me recently. "And there's no point seeking variety where none is needed. Many beginners introduce too much variety—10 to 15 exercises per workout—and their training becomes scattered, and sometimes dangerous."

Perhaps an honorary thirteenth guideline is this: you can *and should* improve your strength at any age.

The program outlined here can be practiced up to five days a week, and should be practices at least three times a week. It consists of only two "big" exercises, and yes, this will give you a full-body workout if done properly. (You may supplement this program with three to five days a week of exercises specifically for your abs—like crunches, leg raises—and low back—like back extensions, back bridges—but supplement is the key word here. Again, the above two categories of exercise will provide a full-body muscle-building workout.) For a much more detailed look at this program, I highly recommend Pavel's book *Power to the People* from Dragon Door Publishing (see appendix for details).

Each day you will perform two sets of five deadlifts (see pages 104 to 105), and two sets of five presses. A press can be the one-armed overhead press (page 106), or a bench press (page 107).

How Much Weight?

As I mentioned before, forget about this idea of finding a weight where you can do 8 to 12 repetitions of an exercise, and where the last repetition brings you to the point of muscle failure. And forget about doing three, four, or even more sets. That's a surefire way to induce muscle fatigue and soreness; besides, there's a better way to get the same—if not better—results. In fact you might find that the hardest part of this workout program is to restrain yourself from overdoing it, or trying to "feel the burn." Believe me, the proof that this system works will come soon enough.

You'll want to find a weight that you can lift—with good form—five times. That means that we're going to go heavier than the 8- to 12-rep crowd goes. You'll want to feel as though at the end of your set that you could probably do one or two more repetitions, *but you won't.* Again, you're not trying to beat yourself up here. A well-executed workout has a tonic effect on the muscles and nervous system. You should end up feeling pleasantly fatigued while also energized.

Finding the right weight may require a bit of trial and error in the beginning, especially if you are new to, or returning to, a weight lifting program. My advice: go light and then ramp up. It may mean a bit of delayed gratification, but you'll save yourself a lot of pain and frustration in the long run.

DEADLIFT

On Your Mark: *Keeping your toes pointed directly forward, stand as close to the barbell as you can. Tighten your buttocks and abdomen and draw your shoulders back and down. Lift your sternum away from your belly button without arching backward. Keep your breathing steady and somewhat shallow.*

Get Set: *Maintain the distance between your sternum and belly button. This will prevent your back from rounding forward (very important for safety!) Press your heels firmly into the floor and keep your buttocks and abdomen tight. Bending your knees, push your buttocks back, as if you're trying to sit in a chair that is far behind you. This will keep your shins more or less vertical. Bend until you can reach the bar. If you cannot reach the bar without rounding your back or letting your shoulders roll forward, then you must modify this movement to prevent injury. You may place the bar on some sturdy blocks to raise it from the floor and reduce the distance you'll need to bend. In the meantime, work on your hamstrings flexibility (see below).*

Go! (Figure 1) *Grip the bar as if you were clinging to it for dear life. Keep your elbows straight. (For the most part, treat your arms like they are nothing more than the things that are attaching this weight to your body.) With tight buttocks and abdomen, and with a strong, straight back, imagine that you are trying to push the floor away with your feet. At the same time the sternum rises straight up as the hips push forward until you are upright.*

Repeat (Figure 2): *After a brief pause, maintain your form as you push your buttocks backward again, bending the knees. Make your descent controlled and deliberate. Do not "fall" with the weight, but to protect your back, don't prolong the movement either. Keep the movement controlled and continuous until the weight is on the floor again. (Use some kind of prop if you need help maintaining the proper form.)*

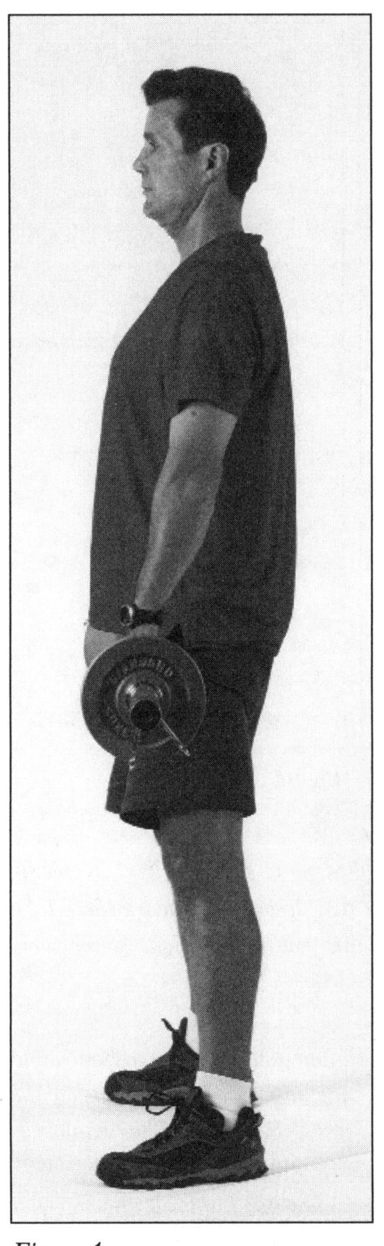

Figure 1

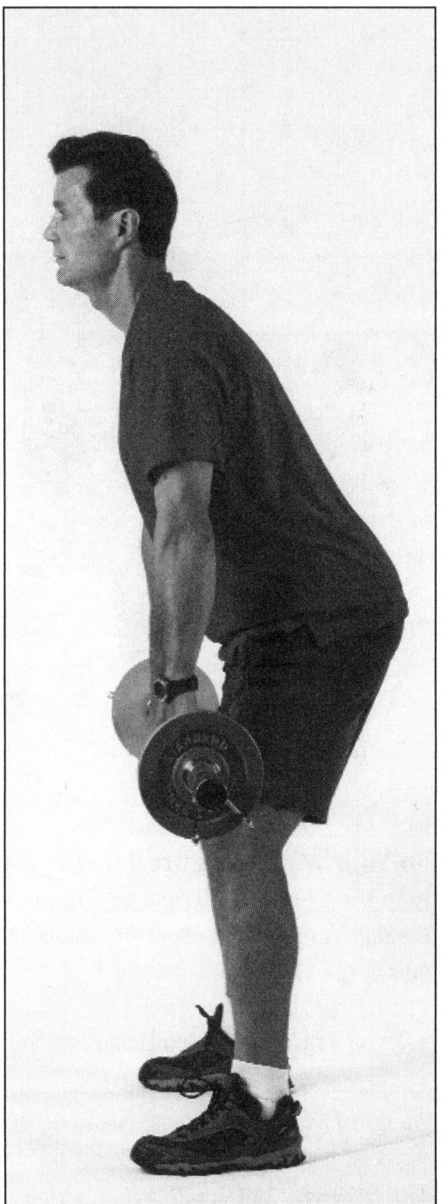

Figure 2

ONE-ARMED OVERHEAD PRESS

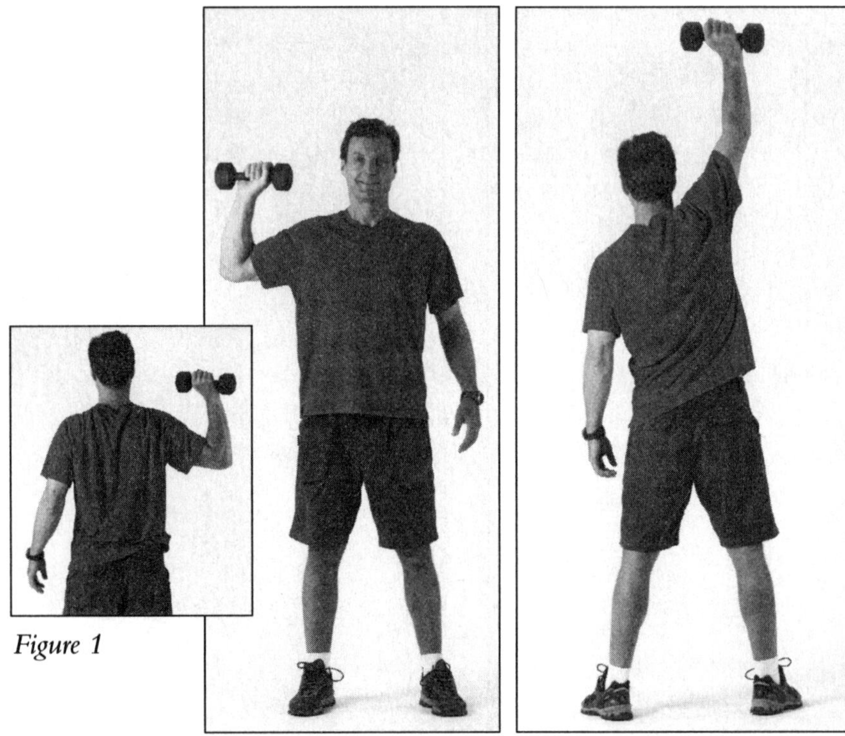

Figure 1

Figure 2

Figure 3

On Your Mark (Figure 1): *Bring a dumbbell up to shoulder level. Remember to use as heavy a weight as you can to lift five times with good form. Make sure that your feet are about hip-width apart, and you have a slight, comfortable bend at the knees.*

Get Set (Figure 2): *Draw both shoulders back and down. (Focus on how doing so not only stabilizes the shoulders, but also flexes the muscles around and below the rib cage.) Tighten the abdomen and buttocks, and put a death grip on the dumbbell.*

Go! (Figure 3) *Visualize that, rather than pushing the dumbbell upward, you are pushing yourself away from the dumbbell. Your body will lean slightly away from the dumbbell, but you must absolutely not lean back or allow your spine to twist. Keep your shoulder down and back, like you're trying to screw it into its socket. When lowering the weight, imagine that you are "pulling" it down carefully and slowly, as if you were trying to keep it from floating toward the ceiling.*

BENCH PRESS

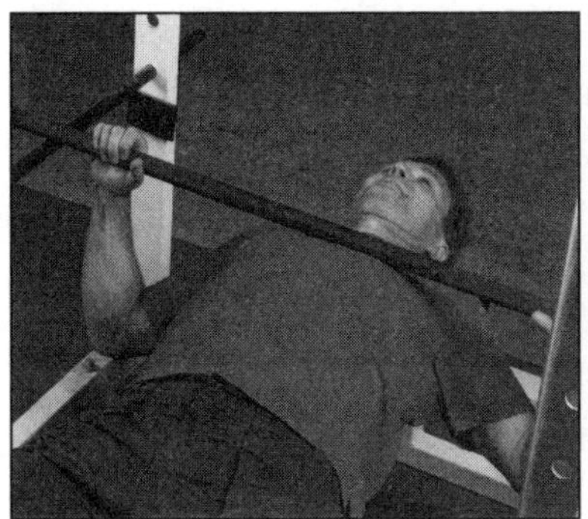

Figure 1

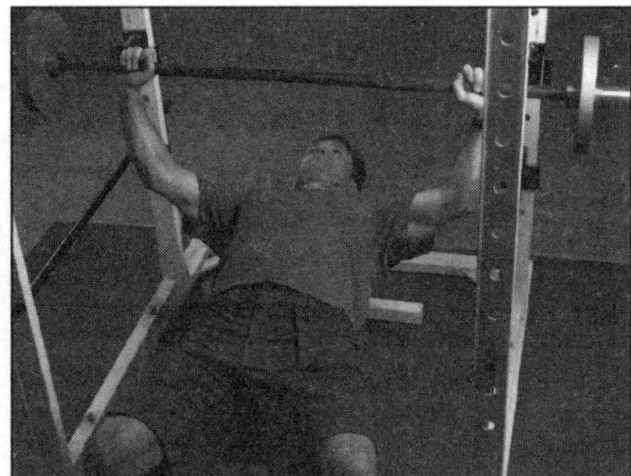

Figure 2

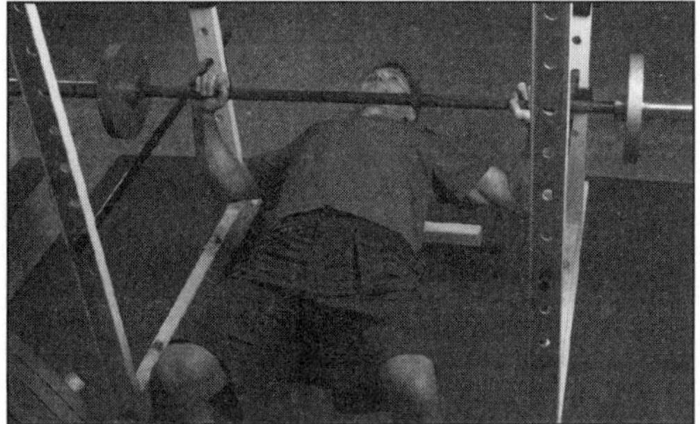

Figure 3

On Your Mark (Figure 1): *Lie faceup on the bench, with the bar bell on the bench rack, positioned above your upper sternum. Keep knees bent, feet flat on the floor. Shoulders back and down, abdomen and buttocks tight.*

Get Set (Figure 2): *Reach up for the barbell and put a crushing grip on it while also squeezing the bar as though you were trying to bend it in half. Push the bar off the rack and position it over the center of your sternum*

Go! (Figure 3) *Carefully and slowly "pull" the bar toward your chest (like you're trying to keep it from floating away), rather than simply lowering it. Pause briefly at the bottom before pushing the bar back toward the rack. Again, visualize that you are pushing yourself away from the bar, rather than pushing the bar away from you.*

Weight Training in Cycles

A lot of the popular magazines and books tell you to find a weight with which you can pump out 8 to 12 repetitions, bringing you to the point of muscle failure. When you can do more than 12 repetitions, then it's time to increase the weight so that you can perform only 8 reps, and work from there until you build up enough strength to exceed 12 reps, and so on and so on.

It sounds like a great idea until you do the math. Let's think about this for a second. We'll take the bench press as an example. Suppose it takes you three months to graduate to a new weight, and that you increase the weight by 10 pounds each time. That's four times a year, times 10 pounds, for an added 40 pounds of strength capability in a year. Let's say you're 35 years old, and you've been lifting weights since you were 18. Wouldn't that mean that you'd be bench-pressing 680 pounds by now?

Show me someone who benches 680 pounds, and then I'll agree that maybe the linear-increase system works. I'm being a bit facetious here, of course. There's no doubt that the linear-increase system does lead to strength gains, but it also leads to stifling strength- and muscle-building plateaus, and life's too short for plateaus.

Cyclical training is clearly the way to go, but it requires a great deal of restraint. It involves considering each of your workouts as part of a series of workouts, where the goal is to start at a light weight, and, throughout the series, build momentum, using gradually increasing weights, toward the heaviest weight that you can lift—with impeccable form—five times. At the end, you start the cycle over again, but this time starting with a slightly higher beginning weight, and moving toward a slightly higher end weight. And so on and so on.

When it comes to cycling, and also performing only two sets of each exercise, here's another potentially big pill to swallow: the second set uses only about 90% of the weight used in the first set. Don't get too hung up on certain particulars. There will be some days where you can do only four repetitions with good form. Sometimes you'll have to round up or down a couple of pounds on your second set. That's fine. What's important to remember is to perform your lifts at least three days a week, and no more than five days a week, and to never exceed five lifts per set—even if you know you can do it.

And here's one more bit of iconoclasm to add to your workout: You can—and should—work out on consecutive days. There's a reason why the high-repetition, push-to-the-point-of-failure crowd is advised to work each muscle group only one or two times a week: It's because after the job they've done on themselves, they'll need the recovery time! At the risk of sounding like a broken record, your workout should leave you feeling refreshed, not fried. You shouldn't feel sore the next day, and you should be able to perform on consecutive days without any problem. Remember that we're treating strength and muscle building like a skill—and skills ought to be practiced frequently. That said, you should never lift more than five times within a seven-day period. Whether you lift Monday through Friday, and then take the weekends off, or some other arrangement, is up to you.

The starting weight for each cycle ought to be one that you could probably lift 10 times with good form. You'll build from there. Below is an example of a series of two deadlift cycles. (Remember, you'll also want to add a press, be it a one-armed overhead or a bench press.) Each cycle is made up of 10 workouts. That's a decent place to start, but again, think "big picture," not the little particulars. Sometimes you'll go to 11 workouts before you reach your peak, or sometimes you'll make it to only 8 or 9 before it's time to reset. No big deal.

Cycle 1:

Workout	First Set	Repetitions	Second Set	Repetitions
1	50 pounds	5	45 pounds	5
2	55 pounds	5	30 pounds	5
3	60 pounds	5	55 pounds	5
4	65 pounds	5	60 pounds	5
5	70 pounds	5	65 pounds	5
6	75 pounds	5	70 pounds	5
7	80 pounds	5	70 pounds	5
8	85 pounds	5	75 pounds	5
9	90 pounds	5	80 pounds	5
10	95 pounds	5	85 pounds	5

Cycle 2:

Workout	First Set	Repetitions	Second Set	Repetitions
1	60 pounds	5	55 pounds	5
2	65 pounds	5	60 pounds	5
3	70 pounds	5	65 pounds	5
4	75 pounds	5	70 pounds	5
5	80 pounds	5	70 pounds	5
6	85 pounds	5	75 pounds	5
7	90 pounds	5	80 pounds	5
8	95 pounds	5	85 pounds	5
9	100 pounds	5	90 pounds	5
10	105 pounds	4	95 pounds	5

Notice that at the end of the second cycle, our imaginary weight lifter made it only to four repetitions of his new weight. That's OK. He was aiming for five, but he was smart about the signals his body was giving him, and decided to play it safe. Either way, his personal best has risen by 10 pounds. In the above scenario, our weight lifter works out Monday through Friday, and rests (as far as weights are concerned) for the weekends. That means that each cycle of 10 workouts lasts two weeks. Sometimes you'll increase by only a couple of pounds from one cycle to the next; sometimes it will be much more than that. And sometimes you'll be on a week's vacation, and won't exercise at all. As long as you're on a general path toward getting stronger and stronger, you're on the right track! It should seem obvious enough that you'll want to keep track of your progress, maybe with an exercise journal, which could be as fancy as one of the commercially available ones at a bookstore or a crumpled-up sheet of notebook paper stuffed into your back pocket. Keeping track not only helps you, well, keep track, but also gives you a nice visual reference of your progress, or lack of progress, both of which are often enough to keep you motivated. Feel free to sprinkle in some inspirational quotations, magazine pictures of your ideal body—whatever works, and whatever keeps you off the couch and away from the chips and beer.

The Trouble with Cardio

Cardio is an important part of overall health and fitness and is the most important as it relates to weight control, cholesterol profile, and general cardiovascular fitness. Done properly, it strengthens the heart and lungs, burns fat, boosts metabolism, promotes a general sense of well-being, and may even help to fight off certain diseases.

Any form of cardio that gets your heart and lungs pumping without putting excessive stress on your joints is fine. Treadmill, elliptical machine, swimming, stationary bike, real-live bike—whatever gets you excited. Aim for three to four sessions a week of about 25 to 40 minutes. And always at a moderately challenging intensity. There are formulas for calculating optimal heart rate and oxygen uptake, but for a reasonably healthy man (i.e., no known serious medical conditions), the old "talk test" should do just as well: You should feel your heart and lungs working, but if you can't carry on a normal conversation, then back off until you can.

However, too many people go about it all wrong, and way too many people overdo it. (Note to all you Spinning class devotees: It's not a religion; it's just exercise.) There comes a point where you can't get any more benefit from it, and you might even begin to see some ill effects. We've already discussed that consistently performing prolonged endurance exercise can lower your testosterone. It can even eat into the muscle you've worked so hard to build, virtually defeating the purpose. And, if done improperly—which is how so many people do it—it can make for long-term trouble with joint pain, and muscle, tendon, and ligament tears. Balance: It's all about the balance.

Flexibility Training

Functional flexibility is probably the most-often ignored area of physical fitness. It's also the easiest area to improve. All kinds of theories exist on the "best" way to become more flexible. For our purposes we're going to keep it simple. We're not training to become ballerinas or martial artists. There's no known benefit in being able to perform a full split, unless it's required for some sport or art that you perform.

Our focus here is to maintain a full and comfortable range of motion throughout life. It probably goes without saying that age tends to bring with it a little more stiffness, in the back, hips, and legs especially. But it may not be aging *per se* that causes that stiffness—it may simply be a lifetime of not paying attention to flexibility. Just look at B.K.S. Iyengar, a yogi who, at 80-plus years old, has the flexibility of a newborn. You can—and should—improve your flexibility at any age. What follows is a simple stretching program that focuses on the lower body. Upper-body flexibility is important too, but (a) most people require more lower-body, than upper-body flexibility, and (b) upper-body flexibility tends to stay intact better and longer than lower-body flexibility.

The best time to stretch is directly after your weight training sessions. Your muscles will be somewhat fatigued, making them more pliable. (And by the way, you may have heard that stretching in a heated room—as they do in "power yoga" classes—will help make you more flexible. Don't waste your time. It's pure hogwash, and it could be *really* dangerous. Prolonged exposure to heat can lead to a sharp drop in blood pressure, and dehydration.) You should try to stretch at least three days a week, which should coincide nicely if you cycle your weight lifting in a program similar to the one illustrated in this chapter.

We'll keep our focus here on the big muscles that can get very tight and noticeably limit your range of motion. Calf stretches and foot flexion stretches are all well and good, but the upper legs, hips, and back are the biggest troublemakers. Before we look at the stretches, here are a couple of stretching "commandments":

1. **You can't force it.** When you try to "tough it out" if a stretch becomes painful, you'll only tear the muscle and set yourself several steps back. Even if you have nothing but the best intentions for yourself, you can't change the basic laws of physiology.
2. **Hold stretches for about 30 seconds.** Don't break out the stopwatch or anything, but go for a semi-prolonged holding time, rather than short bursts.
3. **Breathe deeply.** For our purposes, improving flexibility is a combination of elongating the muscle while also relaxing them, which deep, steady breathing promotes. When muscles are tense while you're trying to lengthen them, it's an uphill battle.
4. **Elongate, don't stretch.** We call them stretches, but that term isn't 100% accurate. The sensation of a properly executed "stretch" should be one where your muscles feel as though they are simply held taut—not stretched, yanked, or pulled. Listen to your body and adjust as needed for the duration of the stretch. (Here's a hint: If it hurts, you're doing it wrong!)
5. **Never bounce.** Attempting to get more depth from a stretch by

using the momentum of your movement won't bring you anything but soreness. Hold still.

6. **Form is everything, depth is nothing.** The goal is to lengthen the muscles, not to achieve a certain depth in your position. You might be tempted to push just a little bit harder so that you can touch your toes—but so what if you can't? It's a pretty small victory if you end up overstretching your muscles, or have to sacrifice your form to the point where you're not really stretching the right muscles anymore. Leave the competitiveness at the door—you'll progress more quickly that way.
7. **Perform each stretch two or three times.** You can do your full series of stretches in a circuit, and then repeat, or perform the same stretch two or three times before moving on to the next. Your choice. If you're going or do the same stretch twice more, it's best to wait at least a minute between repetitions.

SEATED HAMSTRINGS STRETCH

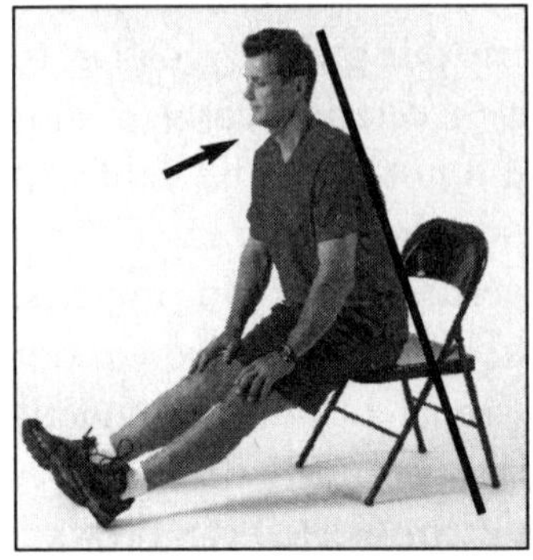

If you're convinced that you have hamstrings of steel, you're not alone. These muscles at the back of the legs are a problem area for almost all men.

Sit at the edge of a chair with your back straight (try not to let your lower back round, with your tailbone tucking under) and your feet in front of you, heels on the floor, toes pointing up, a slight bend in the knee.

Keep your sternum from moving toward your bellybutton (i.e., keep your back straight) as you hinge at the hips. Visualize your tailbone moving away from the backs of your knees and vice versa. To deepen (only if you need to in order to feel the stretch), hinge more at the hips as you make your knees a bit straighter and move your sternum straight forward. Resist the urge to move your head toward your knees or reach with your hands toward your toes. This will only round your back, and be of no help to your hamstrings. Try to keep both your upper and lower back as straight as possible (even straighter than shown in the photo, in fact, if you can). The shoulders should be down and back, and the chest lifted. You can bend your knees if that helps you maintain proper form.

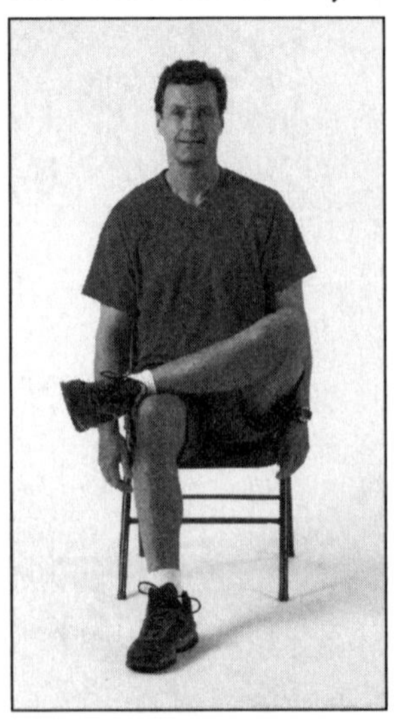

SEATED HIPS STRETCH

The hips tend to hold a lot of the body's tension because they are so instrumental in supporting the entire body during almost all daily activities. Tightness in the hips can lead to back pain, poor posture, and general achiness.

Sit at the edge of a chair with your left ankle on your right knee, and your bent left knee flopping comfortably out to the side, as you see in the photo.

Keeping your back straight (or as straight as you can), focus on tipping the pelvis forward. Imagine your pelvis is a bucket of water, and you're trying to pour that water onto the floor in front of you. You'll feel the stretch in your left outside-hip and buttock areas. Again, resist the urge to reach your head toward your knee. This will only round your back and not help your hips one bit. Pay attention to form and to your sensations, especially to how your left knee feels. Back off at the first sign of discomfort. Repeat on the other side.

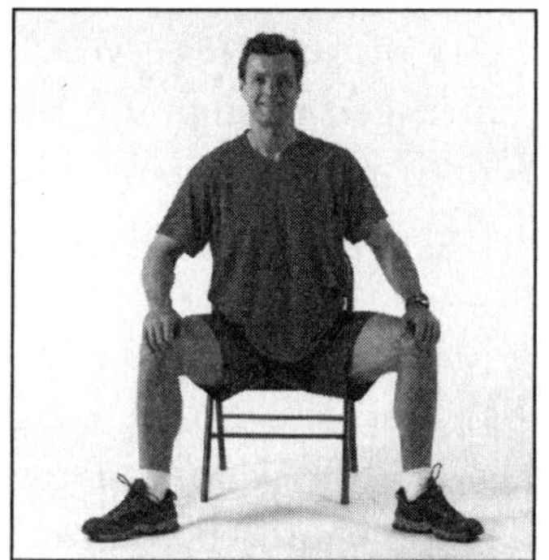

SEATED GROIN STRETCH

Groin muscles are all too easily pulled or injured, and they are all but definitely tight if you don't regularly stretch them.

Sitting at the edge of a chair, keep your back straight as you move your knees and feet away from each other (your toes should be pointing away from one another.

With focus solely on the hips, tip the pelvis forward, with a straight back. You can go deeper if you need to by increasing the tip of the pelvis, or by opening the knees further.

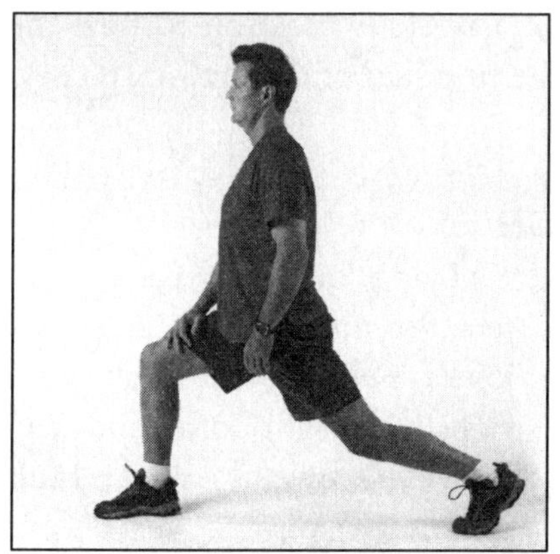

STANDING HIP FLEXOR STRETCH

The hip flexors sit at the front of the pelvis. They're the muscles you would tense if you wanted to lift your knee toward your chest. When they flexors are tight, they can lead to rounding of the lower back, which is a recipe for trouble.

Step back with your left foot so that your right shin is vertical, the knee more or less over the ankle (and don't let the knee buckle to either side), and your torso upright.

It might be a good idea to support yourself by using one hand to hold onto a sturdy chair back, but do try to rely as much as you comfortably can on your own strength. Alternately, you can modify this movement by dropping the left knee to the ground, with or without chair support.

Move into the stretch by visualizing your front knee and your back heel moving away from one another, rather than visualizing your hips moving downward. (Again, don't let your front knee move forward or sideways.) Repeat on the other side.

LYING QUADRICEPS STRETCH

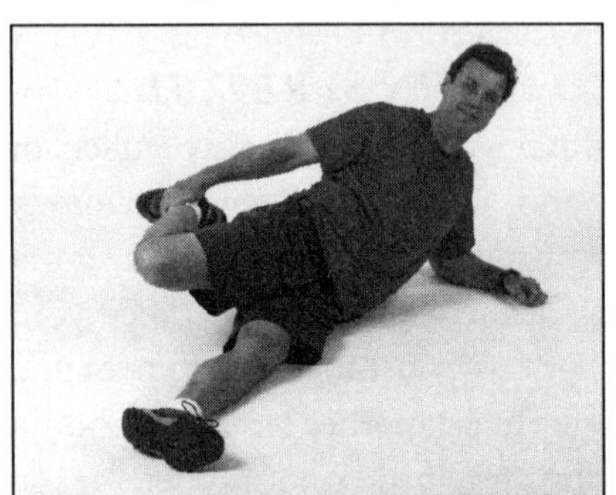

The quadriceps are the muscles in the front of your legs, which usually don't get enough of the mobility they need in daily life. They can feel quite tight at times—tread softly.

Lying on your left side, supported by your left elbow, bend your right knee so that you can grab the ankle in your right hand, as you see in the photo. (If you can't reach your ankle, bridge the gap by using a belt, necktie, or specially designed stretching strap.)

Move into the stretch by pulling your ankle toward your buttocks while slightly moving your knee back. Pay close attention to how the front of your knee feels. Back off at the first sign of discomfort. Repeat on the other side.

LYING LOWER BACK STRETCH

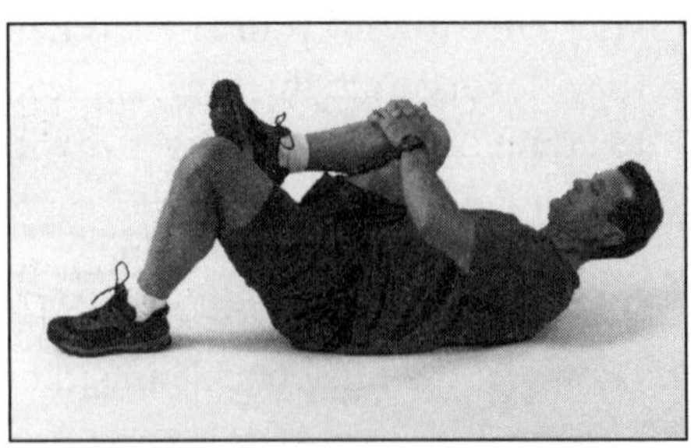

Lying on your back, with feet flat on the floor and your knees pointing up, grab your right knee with both hands and draw it toward your right armpit. (If you can't reach your knee, again, you can use some kind of belt or strap.)

Repeat on the other side. If you can, you may also hug both knees to your chest for a deeper stretch. Go lightly if you've had back problems in the past.

Putting It All Together

Putting together a total strength, cardio, and flexibility fitness program doesn't have to require hour after hour at the gym. You're certainly welcome to go that route if you want to, but you can also see some pretty stellar results in less time, and with less soreness and fewer plateaus. What I've outlined is by no means a bodybuilding program. For that, try *The Body Sculpting Bible* series by James Villepigue and Hugo Rivera or any number of other bodybuilding and weight lifting titles. My aim here is to give you a complete workout to help you build muscle, burn fat, increase metabolism and energy, increase functional range of motion, and feel great—and which requires a minimal time commitment. Try it for yourself. You have nothing to lose, and everything to gain.

What follows is a sample week in the life of the program I've outlined here. (Notice the variety of cardio activities.) Make sure to get in the required amount of strength, cardio, and flexibility training, but be flexible enough to make it enjoyable and compatible with the rest of your schedule as well.

Workout Schedule

Monday
7:30–7:50 a.m. Weight training
7:50–8:15 a.m. Flexibility training...now hit the showers, and head to work

Tuesday
7:45–8:15 a.m. Weight training
5:45–6:30 p.m. Tennis match (and a vicious one at that) with friend

Wednesday
No weights today...still recovering from yesterday's vicious tennis match
6:45–7:10 a.m. Flexibility training before heading to work.

Thursday
7:30–7:50 a.m. Weight training
5:30–6:15 p.m. Spinning class at the gym after work

FRIDAY
7:30–7:50 a.m. Weight training
7:50–8:15 a.m. Flexibility training

SATURDAY
9:30–11:00 p.m. Dancing the night away (the tango, to be precise) with wife
(Maybe a little "extra cardio" later on, if you know what I mean)

SUNDAY
Might go for a walk or a bike ride, but then again, might not

The Low-Down:

Exercise isn't going to raise your testosterone (at least not in the long term), but it'll make you feel—and look—like it did, and besides, it's essential to overall good health. You don't have to be absurdly rigid about a routine, but then again, don't think that you're allowed to get lazy. Here's the low-down: Follow these rules and guidelines, and you'll get stronger and fitter over the long term—guaranteed.

- Aim for three to five challenging weight-training sessions, three to four cardio sessions, and three flexibility sessions each week. It's easier than you think.
- Variety is your friend. You don't have to perform all your cardio on some machine while staring at the wall in front of you. Get on out there and play some sports, go hiking, swimming, cycling, or snow-shoeing. If it gets your heart pumping and it doesn't hurt your joints, then go for it!
- Don't overdo it, but don't under-do it either. You can't cheat your body—if you're not working hard enough, it'll show.

CHAPTER 9:

DIET

DON JUAN WAS SAID TO EAT RAW OYSTERS ON A daily basis to keep his famous libido primed and ready. As we discussed in chapter 7, plenty of pills, herbs, and black-market substances have been around for years, claiming to boost the body's supply of testosterone. But what about regular old food? For generations a host of foods have been considered to have aphrodisiac qualities, including chocolate, avocados, asparagus ("paging Doctor Freud...."), and of course, old Don Juan's standby: oysters. An aphrodisiac isn't necessarily the same thing as a testosterone booster, but it raises an interesting question: What's the connection between food and testosterone? After all, as Mom always said, you are what you eat. So is the burger-eating, protein-shake-drinking guy any better—or worse—off than the salad-munching vegetarian? Or vice versa? If you are what you eat, what do you have to eat (and not eat) to be a well-oiled testosterone-producing machine? In this chapter we'll dive into the always-controversial world of diet and how, if at all, it affects your testosterone.

The thing to understand right off the bat is that researchers believe that diet can and does play a role in altering or affecting testosterone levels, but it's a pretty small one. There are things you can put into your body that will end up either directly or indirectly *lowering* your testosterone (as we'll discuss), but increases in testosterone seem to be (a) typically unimpressive, (b) associated with total testosterone, and not the all-important free testosterone, and (c) usually seen most when a diet is changed to either correct a nutritional deficiency or stop a harmful dietary habit, such as regularly abusing alcohol. It seems that for the average guy, there's really no eating your way to higher testosterone.

But on the other hand, as with exercise, a carefully planned diet can improve some of the symptoms that may be caused or worsened by lowering testosterone. Bone density is a good example. As declining testosterone levels tend to take some bone density with them, a diet with the right amount of calcium can help to stabilize, and in some cases reverse, that bone-density loss.

Calories In, Calories Out

Overweight and obesity are a veritable epidemic in the U.S., with more than two-thirds of all Americans weighing more than is healthy for their height. As mentioned in chapter 3, there appears to be a link between excess weight and low testosterone. However, researchers still debate whether low testosterone contributes to weight gain, or if weight gain contributes to low testosterone. Most likely, it's a little bit of both, and for our purposes, the important thing is that if you can lose some extra weight, then you may as well for your overall health and well-being. How do you know if you need to lose weight? The body mass index (BMI) is a decent place to start. This system compares your height and weight and provides an index number assessing whether your weight is healthy for your height. A BMI of 19 to 25 is considered ideal for adult men and women under age 75. BMIs of 26 to 29 are considered overweight, and anything above 29 is considered obese.

The BMI is somewhat controversial because it doesn't factor in the possibility of high muscle mass. In other words, a man could have a high BMI of 27—and be considered overweight—because he's put on a beer gut, or because he's put on 30 pounds of muscle mass. Professional athletes routinely score BMIs that are higher than those for non-athletes of the same height. However, these ambiguities generally occur only in the 25 to 30 range, and they're pretty rare anyway. If a man is 5'6" and he weighs 350 pounds, I don't care how much muscle he had—he's obese.

There's a mathematical formula for determining your BMI, but for simplicity's sake, just use one of the charts on the next page. Simply find your height in inches in the left column, and move across to the right to find your weight in pounds. (If you don't find your weight in Table 1, try Table 2.) The number at the top of that column is your BMI.

Table 1. BMI Table 1

BMI	19	20	21	22	23	24	25	26	27	28	29	30	31	32	33	34	35
Height (inches)	**Body Weight (pounds)**																
58	91	96	100	105	110	115	119	124	129	134	138	143	148	153	158	162	167
59	94	99	104	109	114	119	124	128	133	138	143	148	153	158	163	168	173
60	97	102	107	112	118	123	128	133	138	143	148	153	158	163	168	174	179
61	100	106	111	116	122	127	132	137	143	148	153	158	164	169	174	180	185
62	104	109	115	120	126	131	136	142	147	153	158	164	169	175	180	186	191
63	107	113	118	124	130	135	141	146	152	158	163	169	175	180	186	191	197
64	110	116	122	128	134	140	145	151	157	163	169	174	180	186	192	197	204
65	114	120	126	132	138	144	150	156	162	168	174	180	186	192	198	204	210
66	118	124	130	136	142	148	155	161	167	173	179	186	192	198	204	210	216
67	121	127	134	140	146	153	159	166	172	178	185	191	198	204	211	217	223
68	125	131	138	144	151	158	164	171	177	184	190	197	203	210	216	223	230
69	128	135	142	149	155	162	169	176	182	189	196	203	209	216	223	230	236
70	132	139	146	153	160	167	174	181	188	195	202	209	216	222	229	236	243
71	136	143	150	157	165	172	179	186	193	200	208	215	222	229	236	243	250
72	140	147	154	162	169	177	184	191	199	206	213	221	228	235	242	250	258
73	144	151	159	166	174	182	189	197	204	212	219	227	235	242	250	257	265
74	148	155	163	171	179	186	194	202	210	218	225	233	241	249	256	264	272
75	152	160	168	176	184	192	200	208	216	224	232	240	248	256	264	272	279
76	156	164	172	180	189	197	205	213	221	230	238	246	254	263	271	279	287

Table 2: BMI Table 2

BMI	36	37	38	39	40	41	42	43	44	45	46	47	48	49	50	51	52	53	54
Height (inches)	**Body Weight (pounds)**																		
58	172	177	181	186	191	196	201	205	210	215	220	224	229	234	239	244	248	253	258
59	178	183	188	193	198	203	208	212	217	222	227	232	237	242	247	252	257	262	267
60	184	189	194	199	204	209	215	220	225	230	235	240	245	250	255	261	266	271	276
61	190	195	201	206	211	217	222	227	232	238	243	248	254	259	264	269	275	280	285
62	196	202	207	213	218	224	229	235	240	246	251	256	262	267	273	278	284	289	295
63	203	208	214	220	225	231	237	242	248	254	259	265	270	278	282	287	293	299	304
64	209	215	221	227	232	238	244	250	256	262	267	273	279	285	291	296	302	308	314
65	216	222	228	234	240	246	252	258	264	270	276	282	288	294	300	306	312	318	324
66	223	229	235	241	247	253	260	266	272	278	284	291	297	303	309	315	322	328	334
67	230	236	242	249	255	261	268	274	280	287	293	299	306	312	319	325	331	338	344
68	236	243	249	256	262	269	276	282	289	295	302	308	315	322	328	335	341	348	354
69	243	250	257	263	270	277	284	291	297	304	311	318	324	331	338	345	351	358	365
70	250	257	264	271	278	285	292	299	306	313	320	327	334	341	348	355	362	369	376
71	257	265	272	279	286	293	301	308	315	322	329	338	343	351	358	365	372	379	386
72	265	272	279	287	294	302	309	316	324	331	338	346	353	361	368	375	383	390	397
73	272	280	288	295	302	310	318	325	333	340	348	355	363	371	378	386	393	401	408
74	280	287	295	303	311	319	326	334	342	350	358	365	373	381	389	396	404	412	420
75	287	295	303	311	319	327	335	343	351	359	367	375	383	391	399	407	415	423	431
76	295	304	312	320	328	336	344	353	361	369	377	385	394	402	410	418	426	435	443

Take It Off... Take It All Off

The benefits of shedding excess pounds seem almost endless, and include looking better, feeling better about yourself, having more energy, and reducing your risk of certain serious health problems.

For all the low-carb, no-carb, low-fat, low-sugar diets out there, one very simple physiological fact remains. The one and only way to lose weight is to spend more energy (calories) through a combination of metabolism and physical activity than you take in through food and drink. Simple as that. Carbs, fat, protein, cholesterol—they're all nutritionally important too, but not necessarily when it comes to body weight for the average, reasonably healthy person. When it comes to maintaining or losing weight, calories are king.

So if you're trying to lose weight, here's what you need to know. Calories are the fuel your body uses to keep itself up and running. If you attempt to put too much fuel into your gas tank, it will simply spill out. It would be great if that happened when you tried to eat too many calories, but unfortunately Mother Nature is pretty thrifty. Rather than discard extra calories, your body conserves them for possible later use, in the form of fat.

One pound of excess body fat is equal to 3,500 calories that you ate, but that your body didn't need at the time. When you put it into numbers like this, then body weight becomes almost like accounting. Every time you eat, you're making a caloric "deposit," which your body will withdraw from to maintain everyday bodily functions, like breathing and heartbeat, and also to fuel any physical activity you do. But just like it is at your bank, when deposits aren't withdrawn, they accumulate—with interest.

Let's say you're not currently gaining weight, but you think you could stand to lose 10 pounds. That means that somewhere along the way, your body stored up 35,000 extra calories. Maybe you overate. Maybe your metabolism slowed down a bit with age. Maybe you haven't been exercising as often or as intensely as you used to. (As it is with most people, it's probably a bit of each.) If you want to lose those 10 pounds, you'll need to "withdraw" 35,000 calories from your calorie bank over a period of time. In this case, 10 weeks would be doable (3,500 calories a week), but maybe a bit ambitious. Let's make it 20 weeks (5 months), withdrawing 1,750 calories a week. Divided by seven days per week, that means that you'll have to withdraw 250 calories a day from your normal intake. You can do it by eating 250 fewer calories, or burning an extra 250 calories through exercise, or something in between. But 250 calories a day isn't much to ask. Most people eat five times per day: three meals and two snacks. Just reduce your calories by a mere 50 each time you eat, and you're all set. You'll barely know you're dieting. Likewise, you could also cut your calories by 25 every time you eat and find five daily occasions to burn an extra 25 calories, like taking the stairs instead of the escalator, or even dropping to the floor for a quick 20 pushups or sit-ups throughout the day. The point is that it's all about small, consistent steps. You don't have to be "on a diet" in order to be on a diet and to lose weight.

But It's More than Just the Calories

Like I said, calories are number one when it comes to weight. But of course there are other things to consider when it comes to a balanced diet, and this is true to some extent when it comes to how eating affects testosterone.

Let's talk first about carbohydrates and proteins. These two macronutrients (meaning nutrients with calories) have duked it out over the last decade, as diet books with competing theories about the two have muscled for rank on the *New York Times* bestseller list. I won't weigh in on the carbs-versus-protein debate, but will say that both are important for healthy nutrition, and as it relates to testosterone, you ought to keep an eye on protein intake.

A diet low in protein may not lower testosterone per se, but may increase the levels of sex-hormone binding globulin, that sneaky little magnet that latches onto testosterone and keeps it from floating freely in the body. In fact, some researcher believe that the best bet for increasing testosterone through dietary means is to eat in a way that lowers sex-hormone binding globulin, thereby freeing up some testosterone. A study conducted by the University of Massachusetts Medical Center followed 1,552 men with an average age of 55, ranging in age from 40 to 70. The researchers examined several aspects of the men's diets—they all ate a typical Western-type diet—and most of the men were overweight, but not obese. The researchers noticed that protein was one of the dietary components that correlated most closely to sex-hormone binding globulin levels. They concluded that "a high-protein diet in older men may decrease SHBG levels and thereby increase bioavailable testosterone."[55]

These findings are certainly not the same as the claims you hear at the gym that more protein equals more muscle. Protein is vitally important for repairing muscle tissue and helping to build new tissue (whether you're recovering from an injury or illness, or are weight lifting to build mass), but there's only so much your body can use. The rest is simply flushed out.

What Kind of Protein?

Protein comes in all shapes and sizes, and from many sources. Again, I won't get too heavily into the pros and cons of plant-based proteins versus the more traditional animal proteins found in meat and dairy products. But as it relates to testosterone, some studies point to a link between the plant estrogens (phytoestrogens) found in soy products, like soy milk and tofu, and lowered testosterone.

One recent study looked at whether soy protein could alter serum hormones in men, and how, in particular, the phytoestrogen known as isoflavone (which is abundant in soy products) may play a role. In the study 35 men consumed either milk protein, low-isoflavone soy protein, or high-isoflavone soy protein. Among those who consumed both the low-isoflavone and the high-isoflavone soy protein, testosterone was "significantly decreased." The researchers concluded that soy protein, regardless of isoflavone content, "decreased...testosterone with minor effects on other hormones, providing evidence for some effects of soy protein on hormones."[56]

On the other hand, a much larger study from British researchers looked at data from 696 British men with a wide range of soy intakes, and determined through the data that "soy milk intake was not associated with serum concentrations of testosterone, free testosterone," and other sex hormones.[57]

For the moment, there appears to be no real consensus on whether soy products can or do significantly lower testosterone in men. At this time, not enough large-scale studies have been performed to yield a definite "yea" or "nay." Meantime, soy products have been widely touted as a low-calorie, low-fat no-cholesterol alternative to animal-based proteins. And furthermore, epidemiological studies suggest that men who eat more soy products show a lower risk of prostate cancer.[58]

What About Fat?

It's not the nutritional Boogie Man it used to be. As far as weight control goes, a gram of fat is has more calories than a gram of carbohydrate or protein. Carbs and protein each have four calories per gram, compared to the nine calories per fat gram. Even so, fat is essential for good health and, depending on the type of fat you primarily eat, some experts recommend that 30% of your daily calories come from fat. Unless you've been living under a rock, you probably know that saturated fats and trans fatty acids are less desirable counterparts to unsaturated fats. That means go easy on the red meat, butter and cheese, and highly processed cookies and crackers, and get friendly with nuts, seeds, and olive oil.

Fat intake has a huge effect on your blood pressure, heart health, and overall health, but when it comes to testosterone, there's no clear advantage one way or another. A Japanese study looked at the relationship between types of fat consumed and levels of testosterone and sex-hormone binding globulin (among other things) in 69 men ages 43 to 88. After the trial, the researchers concluded that "...free testosterone [was] not significantly correlated with any type of fat studied."[59]

Stay Away from Excess Alcohol

You already know that you shouldn't drink too much alcohol because of the terrible effects it can have on your liver and your heart, among other things. A slew of research also points to excess alcohol consumption as being a serious testosterone drainer. What's excess? Anything more than two ounces per day for the average man, which equals about two standard drinks. This amount, of course, varies depending on your size and possibly some genetic factors, but as a general rule, any more than two a day, and you're past your healthy limit. A paper published in *Alcohol and Health Research World*,[60] laid out the multiple ways in which too much alcohol can sap your testosterone:

- It contributes to atrophy (shrinkage) of the testes.
- It acts on the Leydig cells of the testes to impair their function.
- It reduces follicle-stimulating hormone.

- It speeds up the breakdown and removal of testosterone from the blood.
- It may facilitate conversion of testosterone into estradiol (a form of estrogen).
- It suppresses production of luteinizing hormone.
- It alters levels of cortisol in blood, which in turn suppress testosterone production.
- It acts on the pituitary gland to impair release of luteinizing hormone.
- It affects the liver, which processes estrogen. Inefficient estrogen metabolism can lead to symptoms consistent with decreased testosterone.

And, of course, increased alcohol consumption leads to increased fat storage (especially around the midsection), which, as we've discussed several times already, is known to negatively affect testosterone.

But Do Be a Drinker

Of water, that is. There's no direct connection between water and testosterone levels. If there were, a lot more people would make it their beverage of choice. (Sadly, we Americans drink more coffee, cola, and beer than pure water.) But dehydration is linked to diminished function of almost all the body's systems, and it will all but surely make you feel sluggish, irritable, and weak. I'm not going to recommend 8 to 10 10-ounce glasses of water a day. Those recommendations were derived from studies done on active soldiers performing their duties at high altitudes. Hydration requirements vary pretty widely depending on your body size, activity level, geographical location (if you live in hot a climate you'll likely lose more body fluids through sweat throughout the day), and overall health. Simply drink water throughout the day between meals—that's all.

Think Zinc

Strange to think that in a country where the people eat more than any other people on earth that many people are still deficient in several key micronutrients, the vitamins and minerals that don't have calories, but are nonetheless important for overall good health. Zinc seems to be one of them. (Actually, to be fair, zinc deficiency is fairly common throughout the world.)

Don't let the term fool you: Zinc may be a *micro*nutrient, but its effects are big. According to the U.S. National Library of Medicine, the symptoms associated with zinc deficiency include the following:

- Slow growth
- Poor appetite
- Decrease in wound healing
- Loss of hair
- Impaired sense of taste
- Impaired sense of smell
- More frequent infections
- Inability or difficulty in adapting vision to the dark
- Various skin lesions
- Hypogonadism

Of course, that last item is of special interest to us. Severe and even moderate deficiency of zinc is associated with lower testosterone. Researchers studied 40 normal men between 20 and 80 years old. Testosterone was measured in younger men before and during a moderate zinc deficiency, which was induced by restricting zinc intake. At the same time, the researchers measured testosterone in zinc-deficient older men, and put them on a zinc supplement program lasting 6 months. The data showed that "dietary zinc restriction in normal young men was associated with a significant decrease in serum testosterone concentrations after 20 weeks of zinc restriction" and that "zinc supplementation of marginally zinc-deficient normal elderly men for six months resulted in an increase in serum testosterone."[61]

Now, before you go running to your local health-food store to pick up a bottle of zinc tablets, remember that the changing testosterone levels demonstrated in the study all had to do with deficient amounts: testosterone was lowered when zinc was deficient, and raised when deficient men replaced zinc. That's certainly a far cry from saying that zinc boosts testosterone. However, if you are zinc deficient, then a zinc supplement regimen could very well bring your levels back up to what's normal for your age. On the other hand, excess zinc is associated with several unpleasant side effects. In excess, the mineral is toxic, but despite that, many dietary supplements contain several times the recommended daily allowance, which can lead to, among other things, diarrhea, muscle cramps, and vomiting within hours of ingesting an overly high dosage.

Even without ingesting an extreme dosage at one time, consistently exceeding the recommended daily allowance has been shown to increase prostate size and has the potential to contribute to prostate conditions including a benign enlargement of the prostate and prostate cancer.[62]

AND NOW, GETTING BACK TO DON JUAN...

Don Juan's dietary habits may actually have been right on the mark: oysters are ounce for ounce the richest source of zinc available. The good news is that if you're increasing protein as part of your testosterone-friendly eating plan, then you're probably also increasing zinc automatically. Many foods high in protein are also high in zinc, including poultry, which is the main source of zinc in the American diet. For an average health man who's 19 years or older, the recommended daily allowance is 11 mg to 15 mg. While several foods are considered good sources of zinc, table 2 lists some of the highest[63]:

Table 3: Common Foods Rich in Zinc

FOOD	SERVING SIZE	ZINC (MG)
Oysters (raw)	6 medium	76.28
General Mills Whole Grain Total cereal	¾ cup	17.46
Kellogg's Complete Wheat Bran Flakes	¾ cup	15.23
General Mills Total Raisin Bran cereal	1 cup	15.01
Baked beans, canned, with pork and tomato sauce	1 cup	13.86
Beef	3 ounces	8.73
General Mills Frosted Wheaties cereal	¾ cup	7.5
Crabmeat (cooked)	3 ounces	6.48
Beef ribs (lean)	3 ounces	5.91
General Mills Cheerios	1 cup	4.62
Snacks, trail mix, regular, with chocolate chips, salted nuts and seeds	1 cup	4.58
Barley (raw, pearled)	1 cup	4.26
Leg of lamb (lean)	3 ounces	4.2
Turkey (dark meat)	3 ounces	3.75
Pork	3 ounces	2.86
Baking chocolate (unsweetened)	1 square	2.73
Pumpkin seeds or squash seed kernels (roasted)	1 ounce	2.11
Peas (cooked)	1 cup	1.96
Black beans (cooked)	1 cup	1.93
Shitake mushrooms (cooked)	1 cup	1.93

Food	Serving Size	Zinc (mg)
Canned beef stew	1 cup	1.9
Kidney beans (cooked)	1 cup	1.89
M&M Mars Snickers Bar	1 bar	1.43
Ham (sliced, extra lean)	2 slices	1.09
Milk (reduced fat, fluid, 2% milkfat, with added vitamin A)	1 cup	1.05
Cinnamon raisin bagel	1 bagel	1.01

As you can see, zinc is found in foods from just about all major food groups, fruits excluded. Again, seeing how easy it is to get enough zinc in your diet (one bowl of some brands of cereal could do the trick) there's really no reason to become deficient.

Zinc Supplements

Then again, maybe your daily schedule, or food preferences, or possible food allergies, keep you from getting the zinc you need. Then it's probably time to think about a supplement. The good news is that supplements are easy to find and inexpensive. Whether you choose a multivitamin that includes zinc, or zinc alone, make sure that the zinc value of the pill you take doesn't greatly exceed 15 mg (a couple of milligrams here or there won't kill you), and that you don't pop it more than once a day. (Resist the urge to "double up" if you miss a day.) Some recommended brands include the following:

Table 4: Zinc Supplements

Brand	Name	Zinc Content	Price
CVS	Natural Calcium, Magnesium, and Zinc	5 mg	$9.99 for 300
One-a-Day	Men's Formula	15 mg	$6.99 for 100
Centrum	Advanced Formula	15 mg	$9.49 for 130
Nature Made	Adult Multivitamin	15 mg	$9.99 for 100
Walgreen's	One Daily Men's Multivitamin	15 mg	$9.99 for 200
New Chapter	Every Man's One Daily	15 mg	$34.95 for 90
Da Vinci	Spectra Man Multivitamin	15 mg	$22.88 for 120

Magnesium

There isn't a direct link between magnesium and testosterone, but a deficiency in this mineral can make you *feel* like your testosterone is flagging. Magnesium plays a significant role in the body's energy levels and muscle strength. A deficiency can therefore make you feel sluggish and weak. The average man should aim for about 400 mg a day. Again, you can supplement if you really need to (most of the above multivitamins supply the recommended daily allowance of magnesium) or simply pay close attention to eating foods high in this mineral. Table 5 shows some common foods high in magnesium.[64]

Table 5: Common Foods Rich in Magnesium

Food	Serving Size	Magnesium (mg)
Beans, black	1 cup	120
Broccoli, raw	1 cup	22
Halibut	1/2 fillet	170
Nuts, peanuts	1 ounce	64
Okra, frozen	1 cup	94
Oysters	3 ounces	49
Plantain, raw	1 medium	66
Rockfish	1 fillet	51
Scallop	6 large	55
Seeds, pumpkin and squash	1 ounce (142 seeds)	151
Soy milk	1 cup	47
Spinach, cooked	1 cup	157
Tofu	1/4 block	37
Whole grain cereal, ready-to-eat	3/4 cup	24
Whole grain cereal, cooked	1 cup	56
Whole wheat bread	1 slice	24

Testosterone Edge Eating Plan

The old saying goes that many of us dig our own graves with our forks and knives. A well-balanced diet is the foundation of good health and well-being.

Competing theories on the "superior" diet will likely continue to battle on and on for the rest of time. Sit in a room with a vegetarian, and he'll tell you all the ways in which a vegetarian diet is the purest, most natural, most healthy way of eating there is. Sit in a room with a raging carnivore, and he'll make the same argument for his way of eating. It doesn't make things easier that a new diet book is published seemingly every month, and that the United States Department of Agriculture revises its food pyramid every so often. If you know that the conventional wisdom will change if you just give it time, it makes you wonder if what you're doing now is on the wrong track. At the time of this writing, the USDA had reissued its classic food pyramid, replacing it with 12 different pyramids, customized to the user's age and activity levels.

When it comes to a healthful, balanced diet, you could spend a lifetime learning the nutritional science behind what makes certain foods or eating patterns healthful or unhealthful. But as far as guidelines go, let's whittle it down to these five points:

1. **You're Not a Robot.** Unless you walk around with a calculator and a set of measuring cups, you're probably not going to eat *exactly* 2,500 calories a day, get *exactly* 30 grams of protein, etc. So it's a good thing your body is quite a bit more flexible than that. We're looking at general overall patterns, not daily quotas. A couple of calories overboard on Tuesday? Just reach for the carrot stick instead of the potato chips on Wednesday.
2. **Go Easy on the Processed Foods.** It seems almost impossible to go a day without eating heavily processed foods. You might not even be aware you're doing it. They're certainly convenient, cheap, portable, and (arguably) good tasting, but more often than not the foods they're made from have been stripped of their most basic nutrients, and loaded up with sugar, salt, and chemical additives that most people can't pronounce. How do you know if a food has been processed? Here's a good guideline: if it comes in a box or a can, it more than likely is. Check food labels for sodium count and sugar (which goes under many aliases, included glucose, evaporated cane juice, sucrose, high fructose corn syrup, and corn syrup, among others). Whenever you can, opt for fresh, whole foods.
3. **Keep the Fire Burning.** Your body's metabolism is often compared to a fire, and food is the fuel for that fire. Imagine that you're camping and you want to have a fire for the entire night. One way to do that would be to build a fire, and then let it burn out, and then start another fire, and so on. But anybody who's ever been camping knows that the way to go is to start the fire, and then feed a log or two onto it as it starts to die down. Same goes for your body's energy system. By constantly supplying fuel (eating), rather than dumping huge amounts of energy relatively infrequently, you're keeping your body's energy system from a

roller coaster ride of huge spikes and deep drops (think: Thanksgiving dinner). Your eating plan requires—yes, *requires*—that you snack throughout the day, as you'll see below. But remember, the purpose of snacking is to fill in the "nutritional gaps" that your meals for the day may not fill, to keep energy levels up, and to stave off hunger. They're *not* small meals!

4. **Visualize.** When it comes to a balanced meal, it's as easy as drawing territorial lines on your plate. The latest thinking suggests that meals be based around fresh fruits or vegetables. Fill half your plate (assuming it's a normal-sized plate) with vegetables, one-quarter with whole grains or healthy starch, and one-quarter with a lean protein source. That could mean a salad with a salmon filet and brown rice, or grilled asparagus with a small baked potato and lean steak, or even some steamed kale with quinoa and tofu. Do you literally need to separate your foods? Of course not. The general idea is that your meal consist of ½ vegetables or fruits prepared sensibly (fried zuchini wouldn't count!), ¼ healthy starch (preferably a whole grain, although potatoes or pasta are OK from time to time), and ¼ lean protein source (again, sensibly prepared—fried chicken and corndogs won't cut it!)
5. **Mix It Up.** Variety is the spice of life, and it's also the key to healthy eating. An apple is most definitely a healthy food, but it doesn't provide all the nutrients the fruit world has to offer. For that, you'll need to throw some oranges, bananas, blueberries, and pears into the mix. Ditto for vegetables, grains, and protein sources.

Portions, Food Groups, and Meals

I haven't gotten too heavily into portions and food groups yet because (a) this isn't a diet book, and (b) I figured I'd leave it to the experts. The United States Department of Agriculture recently released new eating guides based on its old food pyramid model. The problem with the old pyramid is twofold. First, it was based on the daily calorie needs of a sedentary person. Second, it made no adjustments for age or activity level. The calorie and relative portion recommendations were the same for an athletic 20-year-old man as for a sedentary 75-year-old grandma! The new model bases caloric needs and portion sizes from each food group on your gender, age, and activity level. (See the Appendix for information about finding which pyramid is meant for you.)

What follows here is a one-week sample eating plan based on the USDA's new pyramid program. I've modified it slightly with help from a clinical dietician, Lori Magrath, to reflect the calorie and nutritional needs of an active man 30 to 50 years old concerned about getting the testosterone-friendly nutrients he needs. Averaged over a week, the eating plan provides about 2,400 calories a day.

Monday-Thursday

Monday	Tuesday	Wednesday	Thursday
Breakfast	**Breakfast**	**Breakfast**	**Breakfast**
Breakfast burrito *1 flour tortilla (7" diameter)* *1 scrambled egg (in 1 tsp soft margarine)* *1/3 cup black beans* *2 tbsp salsa* 1 cup orange juice 1 cup fat-free milk	Hot cereal *1/2 cup cooked oatmeal* *2 tbsp raisins* *1 tsp soft margarine* 1/2 cup fat-free milk 1 cup orange juice	Cold cereal *1 cup bran flakes* *1 cup fat-free milk* *1 small banana* 1 slice whole wheat toast *1 tsp soft margarine* 1 cup prune juice	1 whole wheat English muffin *2 tsp soft margarine* *1 tbsp jam or preserves* 1 medium grapefruit 1 hard-boiled egg 1 unsweetened beverage
Mid-Morning Snack	**Mid-Morning Snack**	**Mid-Morning Snack**	**Mid-Morning Snack**
1 cup cantaloupe	1/2 ounce dry-roasted nuts 1/4 cup pineapple 2 tbsp raisins	1/4 cup dried apricots 1 cup low-fat fruited yogurt	1 cup low-fat fruited yogurt
Lunch	**Lunch**	**Lunch**	**Lunch**
Roast beef sandwich *1 whole grain sandwich bun* *3 ounces lean roast beef* *2 slices tomato* *1/4 cup shredded romaine lettuce* *1/8 cup sauteed mushrooms (in 1 tsp oil)* *1 1/2 ounce part-skim mozzarella cheese* *1 tsp yellow mustard* 3/4 cup baked potato wedges *1 tbsp ketchup* 1 unsweetened beverage	Taco salad *2 ounces tortilla chips* *2 ounces ground turkey, sauteed in 2 tsp sunflower oil* *1/2 cup black beans* *1/2 cup iceberg lettuce* *2 slices tomato* *1 ounce low-fat cheddar cheese* *2 tbsp salsa* *1/2 cup avocado* *1 tsp lime juice* 1 unsweetened beverage	Tuna fish sandwich *2 slices rye bread* *3 ounces tuna (packed drained)* *2 tsp mayonnaise* *1 tbsp diced celery* *1/4 cup shredded romaine* *2 slices tomato* 1 medium pear 1 cup fat-free milk	White bean vegetable soup *1 1/4 cup chunky vegetable soup* *1/2 cup white beans* 2 ounce breadstick 8 baby carrots 1 cup fat-free milk

Monday	Tuesday	Wednesday	Thursday
Afternoon Snack	**Afternoon Snack**	**Afternoon Snack**	**Afternoon Snack**
1/2 Ham and cheese sandwich *1 slice whole wheat bread* *1 slice low-fat cheese* *2 slices reduced-fat ham* 8 ounces skim milk	1/4 cup raw almonds 2 tbsp raisins 8 ounces skim milk	Peanut butter and jelly sandwich *2 slices whole-wheat bread* *1 1/2 tbsp all-natural peanut butter* *1 tbsp 100% fruit spread* 1 cup 100% fruit juice	8 ounces cubed low-fat cheddar cheese 1 Medium apple
Dinner	**Dinner**	**Dinner**	**Dinner**
Stuffed broiled salmon *5 ounces salmon* *1 ounce bread stuffing mix* *1 tbsp diced celery* *2 tsp canola oil* 1/2 cup saffron (white) rice *1 ounce slivered almonds* 1/2 cup steamed broccoli *1 tsp soft margarine* 1 cup fat-free milk	Spinach lasagna *1 cup lasagna noodles, cooked (2 oz dry)* *2/3 cup cooked spinach* *1/2 cup ricotta cheese* *1/2 cup tomato sauce with tomato tidbits* *1 ounce part-skim mozzaarella cheese* 1 ounce whole-wheat dinner roll 1 cup fat-free milk	3 ounces boneless, skinless chicken breast 1 large baked sweet potato 1/2 cup peas and onions *1 tsp soft margarine* 1-ounce whole-wheat dinner roll *1 tsp soft margarine* 1 cup leafy greens salad *3 tsp sunflower oil and vinegar dressing* 1 cup fat-free milk	Rigatoni with meat sauce *1 cup rigatoni pasta* *1/2 cup tomato sauce* *2 ounces extra lean beef* *3 tbsp grated Parmesan* Spinach salad *1 cup baby spinach* *1/2 cup tangerine* *1/2 ounce chopped wanuts* *3 tsp sunflower oil dressing*

Friday-Sunday

Friday	Saturday	Sunday
Breakfast	**Breakfast**	**Breakfast**
Cold cereal *1 cup puffed wheat cereal* *1 tbsp raisins* *1 cup fat-free milk* *1 small banana* 1 slice whole-wheat toast *1 tsp soft margarine* *1 tsp jelly*	French toast *2 slices whole wheat French toast* *2 tsp soft margarine* *2 tbsp maple syrup* 1/2 medium grapefruit 1 cup fat-free milk	Pancakes *3 buckwheat pancakes* *2 tsp soft margarine* *3 tbsp maple syrup* 1/2 cup strawberries 3/4 cup honeydew melon 1/2 cup fat-free milk
Mid-Morning Snack	**Mid-Morning Snack**	**Mid-Morning Snack**
1 cup low-fat fruited yogurt	5 whole-wheat crackers 1/8 cup hummus 1/2 cup fruit cocktail (in water or juice)	1 ounce sunflower seeds 1 large banana 1 cup low-fat fruited yogurt

FRIDAY	SATURDAY	SUNDAY
Lunch	**Lunch**	**Lunch**
SMOKED TURKEY SANDWICH *2 ounces whole wheat pita bread* *1/4 cup romaine lettuce* *2 slices tomato* *3 ounces sliced smoked turkey breast* *1 tbsp mayo-type salad dressing* *1 tsp yellow mustard* 1/2 CUP APPLE SLICES 1 CUP TOMATO JUICE	VEGETARIAN CHILI ON BAKED POTATO *1 cup kidney beans* *1/2 cup tomato sauce with tomato tidbits* *3 tbsp chopped onions* *1 ounce low-fat cheddar cheese* *1 tsp vegetable oil* *1 medium baked potato* 1/2 CUP CANTALOUPE 3/4 CUP LEMONADE	MANHATTAN CLAM CHOWDER *3 ounces canned clams (drained)* *3/4 cup mixed vegetables* *1 cup canned tomatoes* 10 WHOLE-WHEAT CRACKERS 1 MEDIUM ORANGE 1 CUP FAT-FREE MILK
Afternoon Snack	**Afternoon Snack**	**Afternoon Snack**
1/4 CUP RAW ALMONDS 8 OUNCES CUBED LOW-FAT CHEDDAR CHEESE 8 OUNCES ORANGE JUICE	1/2 TURKEY BREAST SANDWICH *1 slice whole wheat bread* *2 slices avocado* *2 slices tomato* *2 slices lean turkey breast* 8 OUNCES UNSWEETENED FRUIT JUICE	1 CUP LOW-FAT YOGURT 1 LARGE BANANA 2 TBSP WALNUTS
Dinner	**Dinner**	**Dinner**
5 OUNCES GRILLED TOP LOIN STEAK 3/4 CUP MASHED POTATOES *2 tsp soft margarine* 1/2 CUP STEAMED CARROTS *1 tbsp honey* 2-OUNCE WHOLE-WHEAT DINNER ROLL *1 tsp soft margarine* 1 CUP FAT-FREE MILK	HAAWAIIAN PIZZA *2 slices cheese pizza* *1 ounce Canadian bacon* *1/4 cup pineapple* *2 tbsp mushrooms* *2 tbsp chopped onions* GREEN SALAD *1 cup leafy greens* *3 tsp sunflower oil and dressing* 1 CUP FAT-FREE MILK	VEGETABLE STIR-FRY *4 ounces tofu (firm)* *1/4 cup green and red bell peppers* *1/2 cup bok choy* *2 tbsp vegetable oil* 1 CUP BROWN RICE 1 CUP LEMON-FLAVORED ICED TEA

More Testosterone-Friendly Recipes

What follows are some sample recipes that are high in both zinc and protein. These recipes come to us from the USDA Center for Nutrition Policy and Promotion (see appendix for details).

Beef Noodle Casserole

4 Servings, about 2 cups each

1 lb	lean ground beef
1/2 cup	onions, chopped finely
2 3/4 cups	noodles, yolk-free, enriched, uncooked
1 10 3/4-ounce can	tomato soup, condensed
1/8 tsp	pepper
1 cup	bread crumbs

Preparation Time: 20 minutes
Cooking Time: 30 minutes

1. Brown beef and onions in hot skillet. Drain.
2. Place 3 quarts of water in large saucepan. Bring to rolling boil. Cook noodles in boiling water for 10 minutes. Drain and set aside.
3. Combine soup, 1 1/4 cup water, and pepper. Stir into cooked meat. Add cooked noodles to meat mixture. Stir gently to avoid tearing the noodles.
4. Spoon beef-noodle mixture into 9' x 13" baking pan. Sprinkle bread crumbs over beef-noodle mixture.
5. Bake, uncovered, at 300° F, for about 30 minutes.

PER SERVING:

Calories	595
Total fat	18 grams
Saturated fat	6 grams
Cholesterol	86 milligrams
Sodium	575 milligrams

Pizza Meat Loaf

4 Servings, about 1/4 loaf each

1 lb	ground turkey
3/4 cup	spaghetti sauce
1/2 cup	green peppers, chopped
1/4 cup	mozzarella cheese, part-skim
1/4 cup	onion, minced

Preparation Time: 15 minutes
Conventional Cooking Time: 20 minutes
Microwave Cooking Time: 8 minutes

1. Lightly grease 9" pie plate with vegetable oil. Pat turkey into pie plate.

Conventional Method:

1. Place turkey in 350° F oven. Bake until turkey no longer remains pink, about 17 to 20 minutes.

Microwave Method:

1. Cover turkey with waxed paper.
2. Cook on high; rotate plate 1/4 turn after 3 minutes.
3. Cook until turkey no longer remains pink, about 5 more minutes. Drain.

To complete cooking:

1. Top baked turkey with spaghetti sauce, cheese, and vegetables.
2. Return turkey to either the conventional oven or the microwave oven and heat until cheese is melted, about 1 to 2 minutes.

PER SERVING:

Calories	255
Total fat	14 grams
Saturated fat	4 grams
Cholesterol	88 milligrams
Sodium	376 milligrams

Oven Crispy Chicken

4 Servings, about 4 ounces each

1 1/2 lbs	broiler fryer chicken, cut-up
1/4 cup	whole milk
1/2 cup	flour
1 tsp	paprika
1/2 tsp	pepper
1 cup	ready-to-eat flake cereal, slightly crushed
4 tsp	vegetable oil

Preparation Time: 15 minutes
Cooking Time: 30 minutes

1. Remove skin and all visible fat from chicken.
2. Place milk in large bowl. Add chicken pieces and turn to coat.
3. Combine flour, paprika, and pepper on a plate.
4. Lift chicken pieces from milk and reserve milk.
5. Coat chicken thoroughly with seasoned flour and place on a wire rack until all pieces have been coated. Redip chicken pieces into reserved milk.
6. Place crushed cereal on plate. Place chicken pieces on crushed cereal. Using 2 forks, turn chicken pieces in crushed cereal to coat.
7. Place chicken on a foil-lined baking tray. Drizzle oil over chicken.
8. Bake at 400° F for 15 minutes. Turn chicken pieces over. Continue to bake until chicken is thoroughly cooked and crust is crisp, about 15 more minutes.

Per Serving:

Calories	350
Total fat	15 grams
Saturated fat	4 grams
Cholesterol	93 milligrams
Sodium	503 milligrams

Spanish Baked Fish

4 Servings, about 3 ounces each

1 lb	perch fillets, fresh or frozen
1 cup	tomato sauce
1/2 cup	onions, sliced
2 tsp	chili powder
1 tsp	dried oregano flakes
1/2 tsp	garlic powder
1/8 tsp	ground cumin

Preparation Time: 15 minutes
Cooking Time: 10 to 20 minutes

1. If frozen, thaw frozen fish according to package directions.
2. Preheat oven to 350° F. Lightly grease baking dish.
3. Separate fish into four fillets or pieces. Arrange fish in baking dish.
4. Mix remaining ingredients together and pour over fish.
5. Bake until fish flakes easily with fork, about 10 to 20 minutes.

Per Serving:

Calories	135
Total fat	1 gram
Saturated fat	Trace
Cholesterol	104 milligrams
Sodium	448 milligrams

Turkey Chili

4 Servings, about 1½ cups each

1 lb	ground turkey
¾ cup	onion, minced
2 tbsp	margarine
1 15 ½-ounce can	canned red kidney beans, drained
1 6-ounce can	tomato paste
½	cup pearl barley
1 tbsp	powder
1 tbsp	dry parsley flakes
2 tsp	dry mustard
1 tsp	paprika
½ tsp	garlic powder
¾ cup	cheddar cheese, shredded

Preparation Time: 30 Minutes
Cooking Time: 70 Minutes

1. In large sauce pan, cook turkey and onions in margarine until turkey is browned and no longer pink in color, about 9 minutes. Drain. Return turkey and onions to pan.
2. Add remaining ingredients except the cheese to turkey mixture with 3 cups of water; bring to boil, stirring frequently. Cover, reduce heat, and simmer 30 minutes, stirring occasionally.
3. Uncover and simmer 30 minutes, stirring occasionally.
4. Sprinkle 3 tablespoons of cheese over each serving of chili.

Per Serving:

Calories	540
Total fat	26 grams
Saturated fat	9 grams
Cholesterol	104 milligrams
Sodium	579 milligrams

Beef Pot Roast

4 Servings, about 3 ounces beef each, plus 4 servings for another meal

1/2 cup	onion, chopped
2 1/2 lb	beef chuck roast, boneless
2 cups	hot water
1 cube	beef bouillon
2 tbsp	orange juice
1/4 tsp	ground allspice
1/8 tsp	pepper

Preparation Time: 20 Minutes
Cooking Time: 2 Hours

1. Simmer onion until tender in 2 tablespoons of water in heavy, deep skillet.
2. Add roast to skillet. Brown on sides.
3. Combine beef bouillon cube with 2 cups of hot water. Stir until dissolved.
4. Combine orange juice, allspice, pepper, and beef broth. Pour over meat. Cover and simmer, about 2 hours.

Per Serving:

Calories	220
Total fat	9 grams
Saturated fat	3 grams
Cholesterol	91 milligrams
Sodium	264 milligrams

The Low-Down:

Diet affects almost all areas of health, including testosterone production—directly in some cases, or in such a way as to produce symptoms similar to diminished testosterone. Eating well isn't always easy, but then again, being overweight and unhealthy is never easy. It's your choice. Here's the low-down on food and testosterone:

- Serious deficiencies in some nutrients—zinc especially—can lead to a decrease in testosterone levels.
- Nutrition won't necessarily boost your testosterone, but can correct imbalances that may have been diminishing testosterone production to begin with.
- Some nutritional strategies can increase free testosterone by decreasing the blood proteins that bind to testosterone, rendering it unavailable.
- Balance and sense are—as they always have been—the key to good eating. Ditch the fads and put some more thought into what you're putting into your body.

CHAPTER 10:

MANAGING SYMPTOMS

GETTING *THE TESTOSTERONE EDGE* IS AS MUCH about living healthfully and taking charge of your quality of life as it is about turning back the clock. And any reasonably healthy man can—at any age—take safe, effective steps to stop or reverse many of the common symptoms of lowered testosterone. I've selected the safest and most effective approaches to managing the symptoms of declining testosterone, and left the myths, lies, and folklore at the door. You'll notice the "The Low-Down" at the end of this chapter is a visual reference of all the information we discuss below.

Decreased Muscle Mass

A decrease in muscle mass—and a corresponding increase in body fat—is a typical signpost of approaching middle age. Part of the change in body composition is due to a tapering off of testosterone supply; part is due to a decrease in physical activity and an increase in calorie intake; and part is due to a normal age-related decrease in metabolism.

There's not much you can do about the testosterone bit, but increasing your physical activity is something that just about all of us could stand to do. Done correctly, and coupled with a sensible diet, this can increase muscle mass, physical strength, and naturally boost your metabolism to give you more energy and stoke your body's fat-burning furnace.

Building new muscle mass requires weight-bearing exercise. Theories abound on the best weight-lifting methods, but for our purposes, let's keep it simple. If you want to follow a bodybuilding program, that's fine (as long as you know what you're doing) but it's definitely not necessary to stop or even reverse the effects of aging. You can build new muscle and increase strength by following the relatively simple program in chapter 8, which advocates fewer sets and repetitions, using heavier weights. (And don't forget to balance it all out with some heart-healthy cardio and flexibility training.)

As for supplements that claim to help you pack on muscle, do your homework first before you believe the claims on the side of the bottle. If you *do* feel that you aren't getting enough of certain nutrients in your diet, then a supplement can be helpful. But more often than not, you're better off without them.

Decreased Physical Energy

Feelings of sluggishness, laziness, decreased interest in once-enjoyable physical activity, and becoming tired during activity more quickly that you used are all symptoms of a decreased amount of physical energy. Energy is a complex balance of lots of moving parts, including diet, sleep patterns, exercise, physical health, mental health, daily demands at work and home, and yes, in some cases, decreased testosterone.

More often than not, energy can be restored though simple lifestyle changes.

Decreased physical energy often accompanies low metabolism. Boosting metabolism safely and effectively involves a regular exercise program that combines weight training with cardio and flexibility, and a sensible diet that's low in processed foods that are high in salt, sodium, or saturated fat. And if you think you might be deficient in magnesium, which helps your body unlock energy from food, refer to the magnesium-rich foods in chapter 9 or consider taking a magnesium supplement or multivitamin.

Modest use of caffeine can safely provide temporary stimulation, but excessive use interferes with sleep, digestion and cognitive functioning.

Decreased Bone Strength

Bones tend to become more porous with age, and a decrease in testosterone is among the contributors to this phenomenon. Problems arise when porousness contributes to an overall weakening of the bones, making them more susceptible to break or fracture.

The good news is that you can increase your bone strength and density at any age. After confirming with your doctor that it's safe to do so, take a daily calcium supplemental (1,500 mg to start, unless your doctor says otherwise) combined with a weight-bearing exercise program. Look at chapter 8 for a sample program.

Erectile Dysfunction

Given the wild popularity of erectile dysfuntion drugs, it shoud be obvious to most that erectile dysfunction (ED) is a fairly widespread lifestyle issue. Characterized by a lack of ability, or a lessened ability, to achieve and maintain an erection sufficient for sexual intercourse, ED may or may not be accompanied by a decline in libido. As mentioned throughout this book, ED is rarely traced back directly to a decrease in testosterone, although testosterone does play a bit part. Most often, ED is the result of a physical condition or conditions, including high blood pressure, diabetes, or artherosclerosis (hardening of the arteries), or an adverse reaction to some medicines, including antidepressants. It can also result from depression, stress, anxiety, nervousness about sex, or relationship problems.

The first step in addressing ED is to receive a full physical examination, which also explores lifestyle issues, to rule out the possibility of an underlying serious medical problem or psychological factor.

More often than not, though, ED is traced back to one of those factors. Your doctor will likely recommend lifestyle changes, drug therapy (which may include drugs to treat the underlying problem and also to address the ED), or further medical testing or psychological counseling.

If you have any reservations about taking one of the popular ED drugs, or have been told that you shouldn't take them, you may talk to your doctor about trying low doses of L-arginine. (Your doctor won't prescribe it, but you should discuss it with him or her to excluding the possibility of contraindications.)

Diminished Libido

A decrease in the amount and frequency of interest in sex is a normal part of aging Some theorists point to an evolutionary explanation: After a certain age, it's time to get out of the way so as not to cross swords (as it were) with a younger generation of men wading in the gene pool. Whether you buy that theory or not, it's plain for any man over 30 to see that he doesn't have the sex drive he did when he was 16. The issue is when libido decreases to the point of greatly diminishing quality of life. (Diminished libido may or may not be accompanied by a decreased ability to achieve and maintain an erection.)

Low libido, like many of the symptoms we've discussed so far, can result from low testosterone, or from some physical problem—high blood pressure, depression, or basically any serious disease—or depression, fatigue, or stress.

Currently, testosterone replacement therapy is not approved by the FDA for low libido, even though men who receive it for approved uses do report a resulting rise in sex drive. Working with your doctor, rule out the usual suspects: serious physical or psychological problems.

In addition to any recommended counseling, you can also try small doses of saw palmetto (unless you've been told otherwise). However, any natural efforts should center on (a) addressing any underlying stress or fatigue, (b) a safe increase of lean protein sources in your diet, which may reduce blood levels of sex-hormone-binding globulin, in turn raising the all-important "free" testosterone, and (c) a check to see if you're getting enough zinc in your diet. Refer to the zinc-rich foods and recipes in chapter 9, or consider a supplement. Just be sure not to overdo it, to avoid diarrhea and nausea.

Depressed Mood or Irritability

Everybody feels moody or "blue" at times, but sometimes those feelings take hold and won't let go. You may find yourself not enjoying things you used to enjoy, or feeling sad, irritable, overly sensitive, or "empty."

Depression-like symptoms can result from a decrease in testosterone, as well as several other causes—stress at work or home, poor diet, or excessive alcohol consumption. But depression itself is a serious disease with major potential consequences for your mental and physical health—including a decrease in testosterone. The two are so intricately intertwined that knowing where to begin is often a challenge for doctor and patient alike. (We've discussed already how a drop in testosterone is often misdiagnosed as depression or simply "trouble" at work or home.) The first step in addressing depression-like symptoms is to get to the bottom of them. Perhaps you *are* clinically depressed, and a regimen of counseling or drug therapy (or both) is what you'll need to feel better. Either way, be sure to receive a physical exam, including a measurement of testosterone, luteinizing hormone, and follicle-stimulating hormone. If hypogonadism is discovered you may be prescribed some form of testosterone replacement therapy.

If no underlying physical or psychological problem is discovered, and if your testosterone levels are low, but not low eough to warrant replacement therapy, then you're on your own. The good news is that sensible exercise and diet are proven mood boosters, as is a regular meditation or stress-relief practice. See chapter 7 for more info about Transcendental Meditation and yoga. Other simple and safe mood enhancers include adequate lighting, the smell of citrus, small doses of caffeine. They're not likely to be a cure-all, but they're pretty much harmless, so they're worth a shot.

Difficulty Concentrating

Difficulty concentrating is in some ways similar to depressed mood, as discussed above. Indeed, a decreased ability to maintain mental focus is often a symptom of clinical depression. On the other hand, it's also a symptom of several other things, including decreased testosterone, stress at home or work, lack of sleep, or more serious problems like attention deficit disorder, brain damage or diseases, or Alzheimer's disease.

As with depression, talk to your doctor if you're concerned and receive a complete check-up (including a testsoterone measurement) to rule out any serious physical or psychological problems. More often than not, difficulty concentrating is the result of stress or sleep deprivation, which you can address by—surprise, surprise—getting more sleep (see the appendix for a helpful resource), or "practicing" concentration by taking up a routine meditation or yoga practice (see chapter 7 for other techniques).

Ginkgo biloba or caffeine are at least harmless in small doses, and may be beneficial. Just be sure that neither will adversely react with any medicines you take.

The Low-Down

What follows is quick visual reference chart showing actions you can take for the major common symptoms. For more information on each of these, please refer back to earlier chapters. And do make sure to have a full physical exam, including a testosterone measurement, as well as tests for some of the health conditions that also mimic some or all of the effects of low testosterone, before taking things into your own hands.

SYMPTOM	DESCRIPTION	APPROACH
Decreased muscle mass	Altered body composition where the proportion of fat to muscle tips in favor of fat	Weight-bearing exercise program and sensible diet with special attention to adequate protein and calories
Decreased physical energy	Feelings of sluggishness, laziness, decreased interest in once-enjoyable physical activity, becoming tired during activity more quickly that you used to	Rule out heart problems or other physical health issues. (It may be as simple as getting better sleep.)
		Decreased physical energy often accompanies low metabolism. Boosting metabolism safely and effectively involves a regular exercise program that combines weight training with cardio and flexibility, and a sensible diet that's low in processed foods that are high in salt, sodium, or saturated fat.
		Modest use of caffeine can safely provide temporary stimulation, but excessive use interferes with sleep, digestion, and cognitive functioning
Decreased bone strength	More porous bones, rendering them more brittle and susceptible to fracture	After confirming with your doctor that it's safe to do so, take daily calcium supplements (1,500 mg to start, unless your doctor says otherwise) combined with weight-bearing exercise.
Erectile Dysfunction	A lack of ability, or a decreased ability, to achieve and maintain an erection sufficient for sexual intercourse. This may or may not be accompanied by a decline in libido	Receive a full physical examination, which also explores lifestyle issues, to rule out the possibility that the erectile dysfunction is the result of an underlying serious medical problem or psychological factor, or is a side effect of a prescription medicine you currently take.
		Excluding all other possibilities, and if you're sure it won't interact negatively with any prescriptions you are already on, you may try low doses of L-arginine as a first approach. Or

SYMPTOM	DESCRIPTION	APPROACH
		ask your doctor for a sample of any of the new drugs used to treat erectile dysfunction
Diminished libido	A decrease in the amount and frequency of interest in sex. This may or may not be accompanied by a decreased ability to achieve and maintain an erection	Rule out clinical depression, which can also have a negative effect on libido, along with any other medical or psychological issues.
		You may try saw palmetto, but should likely focus on a safe increase of lean protein sources in your diet, which may reduce blood levels of sex-hormone-binding globulin, which in turn raises the all-important "free" testosterone.
Depressed Mood	Loss of enjoyment in things you used to enjoy, feeling sad or "empty"	Receive a physical exam to make sure that your depressed mood is not the result of an underlying medical or psychological problem, or some other lifestyle issue, including excess alcohol consumption or a poor diet. Low testosterone sometimes produces depression, but all depression isn't the result of low testosterone.
		Depression is treatable through talk therapy with a qualified counselor, which may also include anti-depressant medicine.
Difficulty Concentrating	Diminished ability to maintain mental focus	Rule out clinical depression, chronic sleep deprivation, anxiety disorders, and attention deficit disorder, all of which produce a similar effect.
		You may try low doses of ginkgo biloba, and "practice" concentrating by taking up a routine meditation or yoga practice

PART 3:

This One's Going Out to All the Ladies

For women reading this book, this may be the first page you're turning to. That's fine, because all previous chapters have spoken directly to men. On the other hand, you may want to at least skim through some of the previous chapters to get a basic idea about testosterone. As we'll discuss in the following two chapters, a woman's body produces testosterone for most of the same reasons that a man's does—just in much smaller amounts.

In the section that follows we'll take a look at how testosterone affects a woman's body and what happens when not enough is produced. We'll also cover the current debate over whether medical replacement of testosterone for women is necessarily the best route for those seeking to manage the symptoms of menopause.

Women, just like men, can get *The Testosterone Edge*.

CHAPTER 11:

Recognizing Testosterone Imbalance in Women

YOU'LL PROBABLY REMEMBER THAT THE WORD testosterone gets its name because the hormone is produced primarily by the testes, with some help from the hypothalamus and the pituitary gland. (And a smaller amount is produced by the adrenal glands.) Of course the word testosterone was coined well before it was known that women's bodies also produce the hormone. Just as we now know that men produce a small amount of the sex hormone estrogen, we also know that the female body produces testosterone—albeit in much smaller amounts.

What we also know is that women produce testosterone for many of the same reasons that men do, including these:

- Increased bone mass
- Increased muscle mass
- Sustained sexual desire
- Physical energy
- Mental acuity

Luckily for the average women, though, she doesn't need a lot of testosterone to achieve these ends, and so her body doesn't make enough to produce some of the other so-called secondary male sexual characteristics, including deep voice and facial hair. The difference of course is that whereas men produce testosterone in the testes and adrenal glands, women produce it in their adrenals and ovaries.

A woman's testosterone level rises and falls throughout the day. The level of testosterone that an average woman produces is a bit hard to pin down. It differs from year to year as part of the aging process, and it depends on whom you ask, as different institutions recognize slightly differing standards. For simplicity's sake I'll take the average figures from both the low and high ends of the spectrum. During peak production years, a woman will have a concentration of between 15 ng/dL and 70 ng/dL. Just as it is with men, the majority of a woman's total testosterone is bound to blood proteins, leaving only a small amount as "free" or "bioavailable" testosterone. During peak production years, the normal free range is between 1.5 ng/dL and 8 ng/dL. (Many doctors specializing in women's health say that the desirable level is at about 3 ng/dL of free testosterone.) In a young woman, about half is produced by the ovaries, and half by the adrenal glands. As the ovaries age, the ratio begins to tip in favor of the adrenals.

And just as it is with men, women begin producing less testosterone overall as they age. By age 40, the average woman has about half the testosterone she did in her twenties. However, unlike men, the average women will experience a precipitous drop in her overall production of sex hormones at around mid-life. So while "male menopause" may be more fact than fiction, menopause itself (literally, cessation of menstruation) is a physical inevitability for all women, and a drop in testosterone is a part of that. It's hard to say what a woman's testosterone levels are likely to be after menopause. Some women will drop to the low end of the normal range. Some will drop below it. Others, who have undergone surgical removal of the ovaries ("oophorectomy"), will more than likely drop below the low end of normal.

In this chapter we'll take a look at some of the physical symptoms and conditions that result from having either too much or too little testosterone. In the next chapter we'll go into more detail about these and other conditions, and also tackle the current debate about replacing testosterone in post-menopausal women.

Possible Problem: Underproduction

The decline in a woman's testosterone tends to be a bit steeper through menopause than it is for a man. It may produce independent symptoms, but more likely, will compound some of the common symptoms of menopause, which include fatigue, lack of libido, trouble sleeping, and mood swings, among several others.

Changes due to decreasing testosterone don't necessarily happen during menopause, but they usually do happen around the same time, after age 45 or so. Some of the physical symptoms that can be traced back to diminishing testosterone levels include:

- Significant loss of libido
- Loss of ability to become aroused
- Decrease in sensitivity of erogenous zones
- Loss of pubic hair
- Loss of ability to have an orgasm, or severe decrease in orgasm intensity

We know that these symptoms are linked to testosterone in some way because they can often be treated with testosterone replacement therapy. However, as we'll discuss in the next chapter, testosterone replacement therapy for women is a topic of fierce debate—not only in terms of its efficacy, but also its long-term safety.

In addition to a normal and natural change in the body's production of testosterone, there is another major reason why a woman would see a drop or outright cessation in testosterone production: removal of one or both ovaries. Without one or both ovaries, then of course the female body cannot produce testosterone in the same amounts as it once did. And statistically speaking, some reason for ovary removal is fairly common in the United States.

Ovarian cancer. Ovarian cancer is currently the fifth leading type of cancer in American women, trailing breast, lung, colon, and uterus. Nearly 25,000 women were diagnosed with the disease in 2000, and about 15,000 died from it. Treating ovarian cancer more often than not involves removal of at least one ovary and its fallopian tube. Depending on how early it was detected, and how advanced the cancer has become, treatment may involve removing both ovaries and also administering chemotherapy or radiation. The good news is that, if discovered early, treatment carries more than a 80% survival rate. The bad news is that the vast majority of all cases are not discovered early. Among the common symptoms are the following:

- Discomfort in the lower abdomen
- Painless swelling or bloating in the lower abdomen

- A feeling of fullness, even after a light meal
- Loss of appetite
- Unexplained gas and indigestion
- Nausea
- Weight loss
- Frequent urination
- Constipation
- Pain during sexual intercourse

There appears to be a link between ovulation and ovarian cancer, and that's why women who've had children or have taken oral contraceptives appear to have a lower risk. Researchers still don't completely understand why ovarian cancer develops, but statistically speaking, higher rates tend to show up among the following groups:

- Women who live in developed countries, such as the U.S.
- Women who began menstruating relatively early and reached menopause relatively late
- Women who have not had any children. (The more children a woman has had, the lower her risk of developing ovarian cancer.)

Genetics also play a role. Women who have two or more close relatives—mother, sister, or daughter—with ovarian cancer have a higher risk of the disease.

Hysterectomy. Hysterectomy, the surgical removal of the uterus, is the second most common medical operation performed in America today. In fact, about 30% of women over 60 have had the procedure for one reason or another. Among the main reasons for hysterectomy include treating various forms of cancer, removing fibroid tumors (which are non-cancerous), to treat endometriosis (a growth of the lining of the uterus), and to control heavy or abnormal vaginal bleeding.

A hysterectomy does not always involve removal of one or both ovaries, but in several cases it does, as in those performed to treat cancers.

Possible Problem: Overproduction

The other way that testosterone levels can be a problem for women is when it's overproduced. A gradual lowering or an outright cessation of production is in every woman's future. However, in rarer cases, roughly 5% of the female population, women can overproduce testosterone, a condition known as Polycystic Ovary Syndrome (PCOS), or "Syndrome O."

PCOS. "Polycystic" means many cysts. Women with PCOS, a hereditary condition, develop eggs in the ovarian follicles, which are fluid-filled pockets. Cysts are another form of fluid-filled pocket. The problem with women who have PCOS is that the eggs produced are not released from the ovaries, which gives the ovaries the appearance of containing several cysts—hence the name of the disease.

In women with PCOS, because eggs are not released (or are released only infrequently), there's usually trouble with fertility. PCOS is known as a condition of chronic hyperandrogenic anovulation. "Hyperandrogenic" means having to do with higher-than-usual androgen production. "Anovulation" means not properly developing and releasing an egg from the ovary each month as part of the normal menstrual cycle. So chronic hyperandrogenic anovulation means a persistent inability to produce and release eggs because of the presence of high levels of testosterone. This failure of the ovaries to release eggs starts a chain reaction: hormonal changes usually triggered by the egg release don't happen, and in turn the uterus continues to create its inner lining. The inner lining is not shed as it is during a regular monthly period.

This hormonal imbalance also appears to affect insulin levels, which may explain why nearly half of women with PCOS are overweight or obese. It also means that PCOS puts women at a higher risk for heart disease and cholesterol problems. Many researchers believe that it is this imbalance of insulin that contributes greatly to higher-than-normal testosterone production, and many of its cosmetic attributes. Most women with PCOS exhibit some or all of the following symptoms:

- Acne
- Facial hair (known as "hirsutism")
- Body hair on the chest, abdomen, and arms
- Thinning hair on the scalp

In rare cases, testosterone can be as high as it would be for a normal young man.

Carol's Story

Carol always had trouble with her weight, even as a child. Overweight and obesity were common in her family, so doctors thought little more than to give her the standard diet-and-exercise advice whenever she went in for a routine checkup. Then came adolescence and puberty—or rather, an irregular puberty. "My periods were never regular," she says. "I didn't think much of it, because my doctors told me that it would likely just 'work itself out.' But I always knew that something was wrong." Part of that knowing came from the fact that Carol had a bit more hair on her arms than the other girls at school. It was darker, coarser hair, despite the fact that Carol is blonde. She describes her symptoms as having increased at puberty. Still, doctors told her that it was likely only temporary, and prescribed diet and exercise.

Throughout her teen years, she competed as a figure skater and, in order to deal with the competition, she began starving herself and purging food—the beginning of what would be a long struggle with anorexia and bulimia. Irregular menstrual cycles are commonplace among women with eating disorders, so she thought little of it at the time.

It wasn't until her early twenties that Carol got her eating disorder in check. But that was also when the weight came back, and she started noticing the symptoms again. At 32, she had ballooned to 290 pounds, and hadn't had a single period for two full years.

"I saw four doctors," she recalls. "Every one of them told me 'you need to lose weight,' but I wasn't eating a whole lot at the time, so I knew that it couldn't have been due to overeating."

Finally Carol found the doctor who would make the correct diagnosis of PCOS. Though the condition isn't terribly rare, she recalled that, "I found myself having to educate my own doctor on it."

Carol opted to treat her disease without drugs, instead adopting a modified version of a low-carbohydrate diet, vitamin supplementation, and a rather aggressive exercise regimen. "I knew that [it] was treatable without drugs," she says. Since beginning her treatment, she has lost 90 pounds, and recently had her first period in four years. And at a recent doctor's visit, she was happy to learn that her testosterone levels were perfectly normal for a woman her age. She still struggles with weight, but reports feeling "great." "To me, that's the biggest payoff."

The Low-Down

Testosterone is important for women too, and altered levels can make an impact on health and quality of life. Here's the low-down:

- Women can experience problems stemming from overproduction or underproduction of testosterone.
- Various medical conditions or treatments are linked to a woman's testosterone levels.
- Unlike men, who experience a steady decline in hormone levels, all women experience a steep and more or less sudden drop in sex hormones as part of menopause.

CHAPTER 12:

MEDICAL TREATMENTS FOR WOMEN

IN THE LAST CHAPTER WE DISCUSSED THAT WOMEN'S bodies produce testosterone for many of the same reasons that men do (although in much smaller amounts), and experience certain unwanted effects when there's a drop in testosterone levels, whether it's due to natural age-related declines, or compounded by the symptoms of menopause, or induced by certain medical conditions and surgical procedures.

All of this brings up the inevitable question, just as it does for men: should a woman seek to medically replace her diminished testosterone? In this chapter we'll take a look at the current debate over testosterone replacement therapy for women—the pros and cons, the fact and fiction.

FSD: The Female "Male Menopause"?

Around the end of 2004 a medical term began to enjoy newfound fame and media attention: "female sexual dysfunction" (FSD). This is also around the time that Proctor & Gamble began to seek government approval to market Intrinsa, a 300-microgram testosterone patch worn on the abdomen, and which is intended to alleviate the symptoms of FSD. There had not yet been (nor was there at the time of this writing: 2005) a testosterone treatment created specifically for women. But considering that 20% of all testosterone prescriptions are written for women, pharmaceutical companies have been in rush to bring a gender-specific product to market.

The problem is, (a) no good long-term data existed to show whether such testosterone replacement for women is safe or effective (and some evidence suggested that it is not), and (b) it looks like the term FSD was being used pretty loosely.

Female Sexual Dysfunction is a real condition, just as hypogonadism truly exists for men. But just as it is for men and hypogonadism, many have speculated that the definition of FSD is being expanded by drug companies, who have a financial interest in seeing a rise in the number of people seeking treatment. In other words, a "female Viagra" has been something of a holy grail among pharmaceutical companies—especially considering that erectile dysfunction drugs topped $2.7 billion in sales in 2004.

True FSD affects an estimated 40 million American women, and it actually refers to a number of ways in which a woman can be sexually dysfunctional. Each can be classified as either lifelong or acquired (through trauma or surgery, for example); generalized or situational; and of physical, psychological, or mixed (or unknown) origin. The four basic categories of FSD are as follows:

Very low libido. This is categorized as either persistent or recurrent decrease—and in some cases, an outright absence—of sexual thoughts or fantasies, or a lack of interest in, or responsiveness to, all forms of sexual activity.

Difficulty becoming sexually aroused. Again, this can be persistent or recurrent, and it refers to either a partial or total inability to achieve or maintain sufficient sexual response (this includes physical, mental, and emotional responses) to have sexual intercourse or to enjoy other sexual experiences.

Difficulty achieving an orgasm. Some women with FSD show a difficulty or unusual delay in achieving orgasm, or in some cases, are unable to achieve orgasm at all, under any circumstances.

Sexual pain. This disorder can be associated with sexual intercourse, or with non-sex-induced pain in the sex organs.

The problem that critics have with testosterone replacement like the Intrinsa patch is that it doesn't necessarily treat female sexual dysfunction, but rather treats what is often a very normal drop in libido (which is not, by definition, dysfunctional) brought on by any number of factors. It is, some say, another instance of "medicalizing" normal human life-cycle issues in order to sell a "cure."

On the other hand, you may ask yourself, "Well what's wrong with that? Dysfunction or no dysfunction, if the patch can restore sexual desire and satisfaction, then why not?" The standard response is twofold: First, nobody knows much at this point about the long-term health effects of these treatments for women. And second, the responses in trials conducted so far have been less than stellar. Women who participated in trials of the Intrisna patch reported an average of only one more episode of sex each month than those who were given a placebo.

In December of 2004 an advisory committee of scientists urged the Food and Drug Administration not to approve the Intrinsa patch for women. The scientists frequently cited the findings from The Women's Health Initiative, a massive 15-year study of more than 160,000 generally healthy menopausal women, which had shown a link between long-term hormone replacement therapy and increased risk of cardiovascular disease, stroke, and breast cancer. In fact the National Institutes of Health ceased its study of women taking hormone replacement therapy for fear of putting their health at risk. (It should be noted that these findings were among women taking estrogen alone, as opposed to a combination of estrogen and other treatments.) The FDA responded to the advisory committee's request by ordering Proctor & Gamble to do more clinical testing. (The company reportedly now seeks to have the product on the market in late 2006.)

Who (If Anyone) Should Get Testosterone Replacement?

Despite the current debate over female sexual dysfunction, the fact remains that many women do receive testosterone replacement therapy (usually as part of a larger regimen of hormone replacement) and they're perfectly happy to do so. Risks notwithstanding, the benefits of testosterone replacement are well documented. Not all women who receive testosterone will receive all of the following, but below are the known benefits:

- Increased bone mass
- Increased muscle mass
- General increased sense of well-being and improved mood
- Increased libido and ease of becoming sexually aroused
- Alleviation of some menopausal symptoms
- Improved mental functioning
- Improvement in cholesterol profile: in increase in HDL cholesterol, and a decrease in LDL

Current clinical recommendations for testosterone replacement are primarily for women who have a physiological reason for reduced androgen concentrations, which may include problems with pituitary function, removal of one or both ovaries, aging, or adrenal insufficiency.[65] It's easy enough to make the case for replacement when one or both ovaries have been removed. But otherwise defining an androgen insufficiency state in women, in the absence of ovary removal or adrenal suppression has been difficult, due to the fact that the physiology of normal androgen production in women has been poorly understood.[66]

Lisa's Story

Lisa Hutchinson, Pharm.D., has been a pharmacist for 21 years, and is the national director of a natural hormone therapy program for Axium Specialty Pharmacy in Orlando, Florida. She entered menopause at 28, and had a total hysterectomy.

"Even as a doctor of pharmacy, I was seeking answers for myself," she says. "I ended up becoming a lot more educated than the doctors, I was dealing with." There's a lack of education among doctors, she says, and as a result, many women are misdiagnosed—with potentially dangerous results—as bipolar and even psychotic.

A total hysterectomy depletes a woman's testosterone, as both ovaries are removed. In Lisa's case, she noticed symptoms that included dry hair and skin, loss of muscle mass, and a sex drive that "went from 'killer' to non-existent." She began taking antidepressants to control some of her symptoms.

She began to take testosterone replacement and reports positive results ("the 'old' Lisa was back," she says, and she was able to go off her antidepressants), but cautions that "hormones alone aren't the only answer for these symptoms. Fatigue, for example, can be a symptom of many diseases and things that have nothing to do with testosterone. I look for proof that hormone levels are off before prescribing anything."

But even then, she says, "I don't treat numbers or symptoms; I look at the whole picture." If a woman has lower (but not dangerously low) testosterone, but has no symptoms, then I don't want to rock the boat."

Who Should Not Receive Testosterone Replacement?

Of course testosterone is available only with a doctor's prescription, and in a perfect world, the only women who would receive testosterone replacement would be those who exhibit a medical need. However, even many women who could benefit from testosterone replacement should not receive it. In this section we'll look at the extenuating factors that women considering testosterone replacement should know.

Women who are, or are trying to become, pregnant. Obviously this doesn't apply to women seeking treatment for the removal of one or both ovaries, or the uterus. An overabundance of testosterone can cause difficulties in women trying to conceive, and may also create difficulties in carrying a pregnancy.

Women with PCOS. You'll remember from the last chapter that polycystic ovary syndrome is often associated with the presence of higher-than-usual testosterone levels. It's unlikely that a woman with PCOS would seek testosterone replacement to alleviate the symptoms of that condition, but may be inclined to seek it for other conditions.

Women with past history or family history of breast cancer. Again, drawing from the Women's Health Initiative study, many researchers believe that long-term hormone replacement may be in some way connected to an increased risk of breast cancer.

Women with certain chronic conditions. Because of many of the known side effects of testosterone replacement (see below), it is not recommended for women with certain chronic diseases. Other chronic conditions that could be negatively affected by testosterone replacement include the following:

- Heart disease
- Diabetes
- Hypertension
- Liver disease
- Kidney disease

Women with certain lifestyle factors. Because the long-term effects of testosterone replacement may be an increased risk of certain diseases (including heart disease and breast cancer) in some women—or an aggravation of previously existing health conditions—women who display lifestyle habits that could also contribute to those conditions are at a greater risk. Generally women who smoke, are obese, or live a sedentary lifestyle (or any combination of those three) are thought to be in a higher risk group.

Side Effects of Testosterone Replacement

I mentioned earlier that there are certain side effects for women who receive testosterone replacement, just as there are for men who do. These side effects are not inevitable for all women on testosterone—in fact most of them are quite rare—and most of them are the result of a too-high dosage, which of course can be corrected by a doctor. The most common side effects include these:

- Facial hair growth
- Acne
- Increased appetite, possibly leading to overeating and subsequent weight gain
- Hair loss on scalp
- Enlargement of the clitoris ("clitoromegaly")
- Menstrual irregularity (in pre-menopausal women only, obviously)
- A dangerous increase in red blood cells ("polycythemia")
- Increase in blood calcium ("hypercalcemia")

Testosterone Therapy for Women: A Primer

A full 20% of all testosterone prescriptions in America are given to women. It may or may not be part of a larger hormone therapy that includes estrogen and progesterone, and there appear to be no interactions between them. Doctors may prescribe it alone, or with estrogen and progesterone, depending on the patient. (A certain amount of replacement estrogen automatically converts into testosterone, and in some cases, estrogen therapy alone may adequately address testosterone levels in some women.

Most women who receive testosterone are those who have complained of a diminished sex drive. While testosterone plays an undeniable role in a woman's libido, several other factors can as well, including other physical complications, emotional problems, and lifestyle factors. Before considering testosterone, a responsible doctor should perform a full physical examination and background questionnaire. Every doctor works differently, but among the test or screenings you might expect to take are the following:

Thyroid function. Your thyroid is a gland located above your collarbones, and which controls all metabolic functions. It's like the conductor of the hormonal orchestra in your body. Ruling out thyroid problems is usually the first thing a doctor will do. Often, addressing the thyroid problem is all that's needed.

Lifestyle and Background Questionnaire. As you know, a woman's libido is affected by factors other than hormones, which include stress levels, depression, dissatisfaction with her partner, past history of sexual abuse, and lifestyle habits, like smoking, drinking, diet, and exercise patterns. If your testosterone levels are normal for your age, there's a possibility that other factors are causing—or at least contributing to—your symptoms.

Depression. Depression has a well-known effect on libido. Often, treating depression will treat libido problems as well. (However, several common antidepressant medicines carry the risk of sexual side effects, including a decline in libido.)

Testosterone levels. Obvious enough, but again, the symptoms of low testosterone are also the symptoms of other possible complications. The only women who should receive testosterone are those whose levels have fallen below 1.5 ng/dL of free testosterone. It should be noted, however, that most labs cannot evaluate testosterone levels effectively. It's important to have a baseline, but understand that measuring a woman's testosterone precisely can be difficult. It's a bit like finding a needle in a haystack, especially if levels are very low.

Liver function. Among the possible treatment methods is a pill, which is metabolized by the liver. Oral doses are falling out of favor, based on evidence that they can be harmful to the liver for some patients. If your doctor is considering oral testosterone for you, he or she may want to establish a baseline of liver function before doing so.

Cholesterol and lipid profile. Though testosterone therapy generally improves overall blood lipid profile, the bottom line is that your lipids will change if you take testosterone. Again, your doctor will likely want to establish a baseline.

DHEAS level measurement. DHEAS is the active form of dehydroepiandrosterone, (DHEA) in the body. DHEA can be converted to testosterone (see chapter 7), once in the body. If your DHEAS levels are low, your doctor may try to boost them with a DHEA supplement to see if it has a consistent, positive effect on your testosterone levels. If so, then testosterone therapy may not be needed.

FSH level measurement. Follicle-stimulating hormone is produced by the brain and is a chemical messenger that instructs the ovaries to produce testosterone. When FSH levels are low, testosterone is likely to also be low. Treatment for flagging FSH levels may be all that's needed to provide relief of symptoms.

Typical Dosage and Regimen

Testosterone is rarely a first-line approach to treating symptoms. As mentioned, your doctor may attempt to treat other chemical imbalances or address lifestyle or emotional issues. Furthermore, estrogen or DHEA treatment may be sufficient to raise testosterone levels.

However, when all else fails—and this is the important part—and a woman's testosterone is so low as to pose a health risk, testosterone may become part of a treatment regimen. Many doctors favor testosterone cream or gel, applied to the shoulders, abdomen, or palms. Unlike an oral dosage, creams and gels are not metabolized by the liver, and go directly into the blood stream. Further, there is no sharp "jump" in levels, as can happen with injections.

A starting dose and frequency will differ from woman to woman, depending on what her starting levels are. A reasonable starting point may be 0.5 mg per day for the first two to three weeks before your doctor checks your levels again, and assesses whether to back off, add more, or stay the course.

The Low-Down

Most women who receive testosterone receive it to restore waning or altogether lost libido. But waning or lost libido aren't always linked to low testosterone. Your doctor ought to perform a full physical exam and a full battery of laboratory tests, and have a frank and open discussion about other possible factors in your life that may be causing, or contributing to, your libido problems. Furthermore, you should understand the following:

- Testosterone has proven effective in relieving libido-related symptoms, but some experts have urged caution, due to an incomplete understanding of long-term risks.
- Testosterone is rarely give as a first-line treatment, and should be given only if your readings are dangerously or borderline dangerously low.
- Even among those who do have low or very low testosterone, not all women are candidates for testosterone therapy, as it may further complicate pre-existing health issues.

CONCLUSION

WELL, MY FRIEND, THIS IS THE END OF THE road—for now, at least. Despite what may have sometimes seemed like an overwhelming amount of information, I've tried to keep a couple of simple, practicable ideas at the fore. First of all, yes, if you are between 30 and 35 years old, your testosterone has begun to decline, and there's not much you can do about it, but you don't have to take the associated symptoms lying down. Second, there are a lot of cockamamie ideas floating around out there about things you can do to boost your testosterone, or produce some of the isolated effects of high-normal testosterone, including a revved-up sex drive and youthful muscle mass. More often than not, these powders, pills, and contraptions are fool's gold. Third, medical testosterone replacement is a viable option for those who truly need it, but the threshold of "need" is a topic of heated debate among medical professionals and the pharmaceutical industry. For our purposes, I've stuck with the idea that testosterone replacement is only for those who would suffer serious health problems without it. General improvements in quality of life are all well and good, and indeed, are a part of the responsible practice of medicine. But we just don't know enough yet about the long-term effects of testosterone replacement for those who simply want to reclaim their youth, or address a very real quality-of-life issue that is nevertheless not technically a medical issue. Perhaps in 10 years' time there will be conclusive evidence that testosterone replacement is 100% harmless and entirely beneficial, and I'll be among the first to issue an emphatic "Gentlemen, start your sex drives!" Until that day....

The fourth, final, and perhaps most important point is that while there may not be much that the average, healthy man can do to reverse testosterone decline, he can reverse the effects—the diminished muscle mass, sluggishness, depressed mood, and decreased libido, among other things—with some pretty simple, commonsense approaches to a healthful lifestyle.

Following the diet and exercise program outlined in this book, along with regular stress management and abstinence from smoking and excessive drinking, is your best bet to stopping and likely reversing loss of muscle mass, increasing physical energy, stoking the libido, and improving mood.

We also saw that a woman's body produces testosterone for many of the same reasons a man's body does, but women produce it in much smaller amounts. But that's not to say that when testosterone levels fluctuate it creates much smaller problems. And furthermore, a sharp drop in testosterone happens to every woman, as a normal part of menopause.

When a woman's testosterone drops, it contributes to a decrease in libido (sometimes accompanied by diminished orgasm), muscle mass, bone density, and physical energy. (Though some health conditions are consistent with too much testosterone, the average healthily aging woman typically won't encounter such a thing.) This drop in testosterone is sometimes compounded by women's health issues such as ovarian cancer and hysterectomy, which affect the ovaries, where most of a woman's testosterone is produced.

Medical replacement of testosterone is part of a larger debate on the safety and efficacy of hormone replacement therapy for menopausal women. The debate becomes even more heated when testosterone therapy is considered as a treatment for non-menopausal women experiencing any sexual difficulties. While Female Sexual Dysfunction is a real condition, skeptics have claimed that some companies have an interest in seeing its definition expanded to make room for more prescriptions of testosterone treatment. Early trials of the Intrinsa testosterone patch didn't impress the FDA, which advised maker Proctor & Gamble to go back to the drawing board.

Furthermore, just as it is with men, many of the above-mentioned symptoms are also the symptoms of other conditions that can accompany, or exist independently of, decreased testosterone. Depression, stress, anxiety, poor diet, lack of sleep, problems at work or home, physical ailments—all can contribute to any of the symptoms associated with low testosterone in women. As always, talk to your doctor if you're at all concerned about any symptoms, and be sure to receive a full physical examination (which also includes an examination of your lifestyle) to rule out other serious health issues.

The future of medical treatments is uncertain at best. As more research looks at the long-term effectiveness or risks of testosterone therapy for women, doctors and regulating organizations will be better able to make recommendations or issue precautions.

Glossary

ADAM: "Androgen Deficiency in the Aging Male," a term used to describe a group of symptoms stemming from an age-related drop in testosterone (see "SLOH")

ADRENAL GLANDS: Glands that sit atop the kidneys, responsible for creating a very small amount of testosterone in men and women

AEROBIC: General term referring to the forms of sustained exercise—walking, jogging, dancing—where oxygen is used to burn fuel

ANABOLIC STEROIDS: Synthetic testosterone, which can be doctor prescribed as testosterone replacement in hypogonadal men. (Also commonly obtained illegally and abused among athletes and bodybuilders for performance enhancement.)

ANAEROBIC: Weight-bearing or sprinting exercise where oxygen is *not* used to burn fuel

ANDROGEN: The general term that refers to all male sex hormones, including testosterone.

ANDROPAUSE: Popular term used to equate the age-related decline in testosterone to menopause (also known as "male menopause")

CIRCADIAN RHYTHM: Refers to predictable 24-hour patterns of most major biological functions, including testosterone production

ERECTILE DYSFUNCTION (ED): The inability to achieve or maintain an erection sufficient for sexual intercourse

FEMALE SEXUAL DYSFUNCTION (FSD): General term referring to four categories of possible dysfunction for women in becoming sexually aroused or to have sexual intercourse (or both)

FOLLICLE-STIMULATING HORMONE: Hormone produced by the pituitary gland that is responsible for stimulating sperm production in the testes

GONADOTROPIN RELEASING HORMONE: Chemical produced by the hypothalamus that travels to the pituitary to stimulate production of follicle-stimulating hormone and luteinizing hormone

HYPOGONADISM: Clinical term referring to a deficiency in testosterone that results in health problems, including brittle bones, decreased muscle mass, and depression

HYPOTHALAMUS: Part of the brain that produces gonadotropin releasing hormone

HYPOTHALAMUS-GONADAL-PITUITARY AXIS: The network between the brain and the testes responsible for the processes that result in the creation of testosterone.

KLINEFELTER SYNDROME: A genetic disorder in which one of the symptoms is inability to produce sufficient testosterone

LEYDIG CELLS: The specialized cells of the testes responsible for producing testosterone

LIBIDO: The sex drive, characterized by frequency, intensity, and duration of thoughts or inclinations toward sexual intercourse or sexual activity

LUTEINIZING HORMONE: Hormone produced by the pituitary that travels to the Leydig cells of the testes, commanding them to produce testosterone

OVARIES: Female sex organs responsible primarily for producing eggs, and which also produce most of a woman's testosterone

PITUITARY GLAND: Part of the brain that produces follicle-stimulating hormone and luteinizing hormone

POLYCYSTIC OVARY SYNDOME (PCOS): A disorder characterized by multiple cysts on the ovaries, and in which testosterone is over-produced. (Also known as "Syndrome O")

SEX HORMONE BINDING GLOBULIN (SHBG): A blood protein that attracts sex hormones, including testosterone, and "binds" it in the bloodstream

SLOH: "Symptomatic Late-Onset Hypogonadism," a term used to describe a group of symptoms stemming from an age-related drop in testosterone (see "ADAM").

TESTES (ALSO, TESTICLES): Male sex organs responsible for creating testosterone and sperm

TESTOSTERONE: The principal male sex hormone

TESTOSTERONE REPLACEMENT THERAPY: Refers to any of the number of ways in which testosterone can be medically replaced

FURTHER READING AND HELPFUL RESOURCES

Men's Health

The Harvard Medical School Guide to Men's Health by Harvey B. Simon, M.D., The Free Press, 2003.

A "blueprint" of the whats and whys of the major health issues and concerns pertaining to men by one of the leading endocrinologists in the field.

Harvard Men's Health Watch

A monthly newsletter devoted to men's health issues from Harvard Health Publications, the consumer-health publishing division of Harvard Medical School. To subscribe or more information, contact Harvard Health Publications at 10 Shattuck Street, 6th Floor, Boston, MA 02115 or visit their website at www.health.harvard.edu.

Men's Health Network
P.O. Box 75972
Washington, D.C. 20013
202-543-MHN-1 (6461)
www.menshealthnetwork.org

A nonprofit educational organization comprised of physicians, researchers, public health workers, individuals and other health professionals, which is committed to improving the health and wellness of men through education campaigns, partnerships with retailers and other private entities, workplace health programs, data collection, and work with health care providers.

Sexual and Reproductive Health

American Society of Andrology
1111 North Plaza Drive, Suite #550
Schaumburg, IL 60173
847-619-4909
www.andrologysociety.com

The society, which fosters a multi-disciplinary approach to the study of male reproductive health, exists to promote scientific interchange and knowledge of the male reproductive system.

American Society for Reproductive Medicine
(Formerly the American Fertility Society)
1209 Montgomery Highway
Birmingham, Alabama 35216-2809
205-978-5000
www.asrm.org

A nonprofit dedicated to the advancement of knowledge and understanding pertaining to all aspects of reproductive medicine.

Impotence Institute of America
8201 Corporate Drive # 320
Landover, MD 20715
800.669.1603

Sexual Function Health Council (American Foundation for Urologic Disease)
1128 North Charles Street
Baltimore, MD 21201
800.433.4215
www.impotence.org

A free online medical discussion destination for accurate and unbiased information on erectile dysfunction.

Diseases, Disorders, and Addictions Related to Testosterone

American Association for Klinefelter Syndrome Information and Support
2945 W. Farwell Ave.
Chicago, IL 60645-2925
1-888-466-KSIS
www.aaksis.org

A national volunteer association with the mission of education, support, research, and understanding of Klinefelter Syndrome

Klinefelter Syndrome & Associates
P.O. Box 119
Roseville, CA 95678-0119
888.999.9428
ksinfo@genetic.org
www.genetic.org/ks

The nation's oldest nonprofit organization dedicated to enhancing the lives of individuals and families living with Klinefelter Syndrome

The National Institute on Drug Abuse
(Part of the National Institutes of Health)
6001 Executive Boulevard, Room 5213
Bethesda, MD 20892-9561
301-443-1124
www.nida.nih.gov

A government agency whose Web site contains extensive information and resources regarding anabolic steroid use and abuse

Pituitary Network Association
16350 Ventura Boulevard, #231
Encino, CA 91436
805.499.9973
ptna@pituitary.com
www.pituitary.org

An international nonprofit organization for patients with pituitary tumors and disorders, their families, and loved ones, and the physicians and health care providers who treat them

Exercise

The Body Sculpting Bible for Men and *The Body Sculpting Bible for Women* by James Villepigue and Hugo Rivera, Hatherleigh Press, 2002 (revised edition).

When you're ready to go beyond merely building muscle and strength, and want to sculpt the body of your dreams, turn to James Villepigue and Hugo Rivera. For more information, visit www.hatherleighpress.com.

Power to the People! by Pavel Tsatsouline, Dragon Door Publications, Inc., 1999.

The strength-training philosophies from *Power to the People!* are outlined, with permission, in chapter 8. For more information, visit www.dragondoor.com.

Get Fit Now
www.GetFitNow.com

A powerful resource loaded with news, fitness tips, and discussion forums.

Diet

Food Fit
www.foodfit.com

Devoted to healthy living, this site provides hundreds of free healthy recipes, as well as nutrition and exercise tips.

Recipes and Tips for Healthy, Thrifty Meals

A free cookbook and nutrition guide from the United States Department of Agriculture Center for Nutrition Policy and Promotion. (Select recipes were featured in chapter 12.) For more information, visit www.cnpp.usda.gov/Pubs/Cookbook/thriftym.pdf.

United States Department of Agriculture National Nutrient Database for Standard Reference, Release 17

Follow this link for an excellent free resource: 26 pages of common food items along with the amounts of zinc they contain: www.nal.usda.gov/fnic/foodcomp/Data/SR17/wtrank/sr17a309.pdf

United States Department of Agriculture Pyramid Plan Web Site
USDA Center for Nutrition Policy and Promotion
3101 Park Center Drive
Room 1034
Alexandria, VA 22302-1594.
www.mypyramid.gov

Enter your personal information for a personalized version of the food pyramid, along with several free downloads about healthy eating.

Women's Health

About Women
340 Route 202
Somers, NY 10589
914-276-1400
www.aboutwomen.org

The medical practice of Jennifer Landa, M.D., (mentioned in this book)

Healthy Women, Healthy Lives by Susan E. Hankinson, R.N., Sc.D., Graham A. Colditz, M.D., JoAnn E. Manson, M.D., and Frank E. Speizer, M.D., Fireside, 2001.

A reference book to women's health issue based on research from the Harvard Medical School Nurses' Health Study.

References

[1] Levey, Collin. "It's About Terrorism, John, Not Testosterone Levels," *The Seattle Times,* October 22, 2004.

[2] Glass, Ira (host). "Testosterone," *This American Life,* Episode 220, originally aired August 30, 2002.

[3] Sapolsky, Robert M. *Why Zebras Don't Get Ulcers: An Updated Guide to Stress, Stress-Related Diseases, and Coping.* New York: W.H. Freeman and Company, 1994.

[4] Kassin, Saul. *Psychology.* Boston: Houghton Mifflin Company, 1995.

[5] Bussiere, Joseph. "Androgen Ablation Impairs Hippocampal-dependent Verbal Memory Processes," Presented to the Society for Neuroscience, San Diego, CA, October 24, 2004.

[6] Shores, Molly M. et al. "Increased Incidence of Diagnosed Depressive Illness in Hypogonadal Older Men," *Archives of General Psychiatry,* 61(2); 112–208, February 2004.

[7] Hershman, Tania. "Watching Brain Waves Could Quantify Libido," NewScientist (electronic edition), January, 2005.

[8] Dabbs JM Jr, et al. "Saliva Testosterone and Criminal Violence in Young Adult Prison Inmates." *Psychosomatic Medicine,* 49(2):174–82, March-April, 1987.

[9] Dabbs JM Jr, et al. "Salivary Testosterone and Cortisol Among Late Adolescent Male Offenders," *Journal of Abnormal Child Psychology,* 19(4):469-78, August 1991.

[10] Bernhardt, Paul C. et al. "Testosterone Changes During Vicarious Experiences of Winning and Losing Among Fans at Sporting Events," *Physiology and Behavior,* 65(1): 59–62, August 1998.

[11] Mental Health Business Week, "Oregon Health & Science University; Testosterone Deprivation Makes Men Forget," November 20, 2004

[12] Roden, et al. "Augmentation of T Cell Levels and Responses Induced by Androgen Deprivation," *The Journal of Immunology*, November 15, 2004.

[13] Dabbs JM Jr. "Salivary Testosterone Measurements: Collecting, Storing, and Mailing Saliva Samples," *Physiology & Behavior,* 49(4):815–7, April, 1991.

[14] Dhindsa S, et al. "Frequent Occurrence of Hypogonadotropic Hypogonadism in Type 2 Diabetes," *Journal of Clinical Endocrinology,* 89(11):5462-8, November, 2004.

[15] Nilsson PM, et al. "Adverse Effects of Psychosocial Stress on Gonadal Function and Insulin Levels in Middle-aged Males," *Journal of Internal Medicine,* 237(5):479–86, May, 1995.

[16] Svartberg J, et al. "Waist Circumference and Testosterone Levels in Community Dwelling Men. The Tromso Study," *European Journal of Epidemiology,* 19(7):657–63, 2004.

[17] Longcope et al. "Diet and Sex Hormone-Binding Globulin," *Journal of Clinical Endocrinology & Metabolism,* 2000; 85(Jan.):293–6.

[18] Burnham, et al. "Men in Committed Relationships Have Lower Testosterone," *Hormones and Behavior,* volume 44, Issue 2 , August 2003, Pages 119–122

[19] Rosario, Emily R., MS. et al. "Age-Related Testosterone Depletion and the Development of Alzheimer Disease," *The Journal of the American Medical Association,* Volume 292(12), 22/29 September 2004, p 1431–1432.

[20] Shores MM, et al. "Increased Incidence of Diagnosed Depressive Illness in Hypogonadal Older Men," *Archives of General Psychiatry*, 2004 Feb;61(2):162–7.

[21] Bhasin, Shalender MD; Herbst, Karen MD, PHD. "Testosterone and Atherosclerosis Progression in Men," *Diabetes Care,* Volume 26(6), June 2003, pp 1929–1931.

[22] James, William H. "Further Evidence That Low Androgen Values Are a Cause of Rheumatoid Arthritis: The Response of Rheumatoid Arthritis to Seriously Stressful Life Events," *Annals of Rheumatic Disease,* September 1997;56:566–567.

[23] Heller CG and Myers G. "The Male Climacteric, Its Symptomatology, Diagnosis and Treatment," *Journal of the American Medical Association* 1944; 126(8):472–477.

[24] "Is There a 'Male Menopause'—and Will Hormones Help?" *Harvard Men's Health Watch,* June 2004.

[25] IMS report, "The Extent and Nature of Testosterone Use," 2003.

[26] Mayo Clinic Staff, "Testosterone Therapy: The Answer for Aging Men?" April 13, 2004.

[27] T Liverman, Catharyn and Dan G Blazer, Editors. "Testosterone and Aging: Clinical Research Directions," Board on Health Sciences Policy, Institute of Medicine, 2004.

[28] The National Institute on Aging, Press release, "NIA Statement on IOM Testosterone Report," November 12, 2003.

[29] "Hormone Replacement, the Male Version," *Harvard Health Letter,* May, 2004.

[30] Simon, Harvey B, M.D. *The Harvard Medical School's Guide to Men's Health,* New York: The Free Press, 2002

[31] "Risks of Testosterone-Replacement Therapy and Recommendations for Monitoring," *New England Journal of Medicine,* 2004, 350: 482–92.

[32] Pope, Harrison G., Jr., M.D., et al. "Testosterone Gel Supplementation for Men With Refractory Depression: A Randomized, Placebo-Controlled Trial," American Journal of Psychiatry, 160:105–111, January 2003

[33] Brown, Gregory A, et al. "Effect of Oral DHEA on Serum Testosterone and Adaptations to Resistance Training in Young Men," *Journal of Applied Physiology,* Vol. 87, Issue 6, 2274–2283, December 1999.

[34] Editorial, "Muscle Flexing in Congress," *The New York Times,* April 20, 2005.

[35] Hatch, Orrin. "Why DHEA Isn't Banned: A View from the Senate," Letter to the Editor, *The New York Times,* April 27, 2005.

[36] Antonio J, et al. "The Effects of Tribulus Terrestris on Body Composition and Exercise Performance in Resistance-Trained Males," *International Journal of Sport Nutrition and Exercise Metabolism* 10(2):208–15, June 2000.

[37] Brilla, L R and Conte, V. "Effects of a Novel Zinc-Magnesium Formulation on Hormones and Strength," *Journal of Exercise Physiology,* Vol 3, No. 4, October 2000.

[38] Gambelunghe C, et al. "Effects of Chrysin on Urinary Testosterone Levels in Human Males," *Journal of Medical Food,* 6(4): 387–90, Winter, 2003.

[39] Schottner M, et al. "Lignans from the Roots of Urtica Dioica and their Metabolites Bind to Human Sex Hormone Binding Globulin (SHBG)," *Planta Medicine,* 63(6):529–32, December, 1997.

[40] Ang HH, et al. "Effects of Eurycoma longifolia Jack on Sexual Qualities in Middle aged Male Rats," *Phytomedicine,* 10(6-7):590–3, 2003.

[41] Ito T, Kawahara, et al. "The Effects of ArginMax, a Natural Dietary Supplement for Enhancement of Male Sexual Function," Hawaii Medical Journal, 57(12):741–4, December, 1998.

[42] Lebret T, et al. "Efficacy and Safety of a Novel Combination of L-arginine Glutamate and Yohimbine Hydrochloride: A New Oral Therapy for Erectile Dysfunction," *European Urology,* 41(6): 608-13, June, 2002.

[43] Cieza A, Maier P, Poppel E. "Effects of Ginkgo Biloba on Mental Functioning in Healthy Volunteers," *Archives of Medical Research,* 34(5):373–81; September-October, 2003.

[44] Haskell CF, et al. "Cognitive and Mood Improvements of Caffeine in Habitual Consumers and Habitual Non-consumers of Caffeine," *Psychopharmacology,* 179(4):813–25, January 28, 2005.

[45] Barnes P, et al. "CDC Advance Data Report #343, Complementary and Alternative Medicine Use Among Adults: United States, 2002," May 27, 2004.

[46] MacLean CR, et al. "Effects of the Transcendental Meditation Program on Adaptive Mechanisms: Changes in Hormone Levels and Responses to Stress after 4 Months of Practice," *Psychoneuroendocrinology,* 22(4):277–95, May 1997.

[47] Yoon IY, et al. "Luteinizing Hormone Following Light Exposure in Healthy Young Men," *Neuroscience Letters,* 24;341(1):25–8, April, 2003.

[48] Kho HG, et al. "The Use of Acupuncture in the Treatment of Erectile Dysfunction," *International Journal of Impotence Research,* 11(1):41–6, February, 1999.

[49] King, AC, et al. "Moderate-intensity Exercise and Self-rated Quality of Sleep in Older Adults: A Randomized, Controlled Trial," *Journal of the American Medical Association,* 277(1): 32–37, January 1997.

[50] Vogel, RB et al. "Increase of Free and Total Testosterone During Submaximal Exercise in Normal Males," *Medicine & Science in Sports & Exercise,* 17(1): 119–23, February, 1985.

[51] Izquierdo, M et al. "Effects of Strength Training on Muscle Power and Serum Hormones in Middle-aged and Older Men," *Journal of Applied Physiology,* 90(4): 1497–1507, April 2001.

[52] Hackney, AC et al. "Basal Testicular Testosterone Production in Endurance-trained Men is Suppressed," *European Journal of Applied Physiology,* 89(2): 198–201, April, 2003.

[53] "The Numbers Count: Mental Disorders in America: A summary of statistics describing the prevalence of mental disorders in America," The National Institute of Mental Health, 2001.

[54] Blumenthal, James H., Ph.D., et al. "Effects of Exercise Training on Older Adults with Major Depression," *Archives of Internal Medicine,* 159(19): October 25, 1999.

[55] Longcope C., et al. "Eating a Low-protein Diet May Contribute to Low Testosterone Levels and Bone Loss in Older Men," *Geriatrics,* 55(4); 84; April, 2000.

[56] Dillingham BL, et al. "Soy Protein Isolates ofVarying Isoflavone Content Exert Minor Effects on Serum Reproductive Hormones in Healthy Young Men," *Journal of Nutrition,* 135(3):584-91, March 2005.

[57] Allen, NE et al. "Soy Milk Intake in Relation to Serum Sex Hormones in British Men," *Nutrition and Cancer,* 41(1–2); 41-6, 2001.

[58] Hussain M, et al. "Soy Isoflavones in the Treatment of Prostate Cancer," *Nutrition and Cancer,* 47(2):111–7; 2003.

[59] Nagata C, et al. "Relationships Between Types of Fat Consumed and Serum Estrogen and Androgen Concentrations in Japanese Men," *Nutrition and Cancer,* 38(2):163–7; 2000.

[60] Emanuele, Mary Ann, Emanuele, Nicholas V. "Alcohol's Effects on Male Reproduction," *Alcohol Health & Research World,* 22(3); 0090–838X, September 1, 1998.

[61] Prasad, Ananda, et al. "Zinc Status and Serum Testosterone Levels of Healthy Adults," *Nutrition,* 12:344–348, 1996.

[62] Moyad MA. "Zinc for Prostate Disease and other Conditions: A Little Evidence, a Lot of Hype, and a Significant Potential Problem," Urologic Nursing. 24(1):49–52; February 2004.

[63] United States Department of Agriculture, "National Nutrient Database for Standard Reference," Release 17.

[64] USDA Nutrient Database for Standard References, Release 15

[65] Shifren, JL, "The Role of Androgens in Female Sexual Dysfunction," *Mayo Clinic Proceedings,* 79(4 Suppl): S19–24, April 2004.

[66] Chu, MC, Lobo, RA. "Formulations and Use of Androgens in Women," *Mayo Clinic Proceedings,* 79(4 Suppl):S3–7, April, 2004

INDEX

About the Author

Brian E. O'Neill is an award-winning writer and speaker. The New England chapter of the American Medical Writers Association awarded the hardcover edition of *The Testosterone Edge* a 2006 Will Solemine Award for Excellence in Medical Communication. He is a co-author of *The Harvard Medical School Guide to Lowering Your Blood Pressure*, (with Herbert Benson, M.D., and Aggie Casey, R.N., McGraw-Hill, 2006).

Formerly editor-in-chief of the award-winning *Working Nights* publications series, Brian is currently a senior communications specialist for a large health care organization. He maintains a diverse portfolio of private clients, including Harvard Medical School, the IDEA Health and Fitness Association, Healthcare Middle East, and many others.

Brian regularly speaks to, and leads workshops for, professional organizations, aspiring writers, and youth groups about writing and communications. He is frequently quoted in the press, including *The New York Times*, *The Boston Herald*, and the CBS Radio Network. He lives in Boston with his wife. Contact Brian at brian@brianeoneill.com or www.brianeoneill.com.